AF597486

Managing Change
Changing Medicine

Dedicated to Mary Alice Parr

Managing Change
Changing Medicine

PARK NICOLLET
75 YEARS

James R. Hare, Jr.

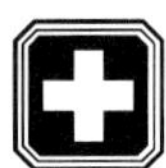

PARK NICOLLET PRESS
Minneapolis

Park Nicollet Press
Institute for Research and Education
3800 Park Nicollet Boulevard
Minneapolis, Minnesota 55416-2699

Library of Congress Cataloging-in-Publication Data
Hare, James R., Jr.
Managing change, changing medicine: Park Nicollet 75 years / James R. Hare, Jr.
p. cm
includes index.
ISBN 0-9655104-0-9
1. Park Nicollet Medical Center (Minneapolis, Minn.) — History. 2. Nicollet Clinic — History. 3. St. Louis Park Medical Center — History. I . Title.
RA982.M6P374 1996
362,1'2'09776579 — dc21 96-37059
CIP

Cover Design Studio Artz
Text Design Nora Koch
Editorial Director Karol Carstensen
Associate Editor Judy Peacock
Production Manager Gail Devery

Printed in the United States of America

Table of Contents

ACKNOWLEDGEMENTS

Writing a first book is a wonderful and terrifying experience. Capturing the life of an organization through an oral history project is more work, and more fun, than I could have imagined. Literally hundreds of people have made contributions, though none more than Jim Toscano, who conceived the project and defended it through its long gestation. Stuart Hanson and James Reinertsen helped with hours of interviews and guidance in understanding the medical marketplace as it was and is. Karol Carstensen and Judy Peacock made sure the words on the page bore a passing resemblance to what I meant to say.

Robert "Bud" Green, Arnold Anderson, Howard Horns, Richard Migliori and many others gave generously of their time. Robert Newell and William Costello both took a great interest in the project although, sadly, Bob only lived to see the first section. Special thanks go to all sixty plus people who shared their time, their wit, their memories, their files and sometimes their coffee during our two to three hour talks. Thanks too to Deborah Westlund at Northern Counties Secretarial Services, whose transcription skills made reliving the transcripts a pleasure, and to all the administration and accounting staffs at the Institute for Research and Education and Park Nicollet Clinic, who always made me feel welcome when I came poking around looking for another obscure and long forgotten article. Thanks especially to my wife Becky Glass, who never tired of her role as first reader.

James R. Hare, Jr.

A special thanks to the following people who were interviewed during the development of this book:

Donald J. Abrams, M.D.
Don P. Amren, M.D.
Arnold S. Anderson, M.D.
David M. Anderson, M.D.
Elaine S. Anderson
J. Roger Asplin
Melvin P. Baken, Jr., M.D.
Phyllis Barno
Paul B. Batalden, M.D.
Northrop Beach, M.D.
Robert B. Benjamin, M.D.
Rueben Berman, M.D.
Max A. Boller, M.D.
A. Charles Bredesen
Marjorie E. Canning, R.N.
William E. Costello
Rosemary Dorion, R.N.
Rodney R. Dueck, M.D.
Paul M. Ellwood, Jr., M.D.
Fredrick W. Engstrom, M.D.
Ruth Erickson, R.N.
Donnell D. Etzwiler, M.D.
William R. Fifer, M.D.
Donald W. Freeman, M.D.
William G. Gamble, M.D.
Dorothy Goodspeed Gale, R.N.
Robert A. Green, M.D.
George C. Halvorson
A. Stuart Hanson, M.D.
Carol Hersman, R.N.
Tom W. Hobban
Howard L. Horns, M.D.
Arthur W. Ide, Jr., M.D.
Charles L. Jacobson, M.D.
Wyman E. Jacobson, M.D.
David A. Jensen
Frank E. Johnson, M.D.
John W. LaBree, M.D.
George W. Lund, M.D.
Donald L. Madison, M.D.
Nicholas M. Mensheha, M.D.
Richard J. Migliori, M.D.
Joseph W. Mitlyng
Clinton Morrison
A. James Neilson
Glen D. Nelson, M.D.
Robert L. Newell
J. Paul O'Connor
Mario A. Petrini, M.D.
Leslie Pratt, M.D.
Harley J. Racer, M.D.
Thomas M. Recht, M.D.
James L. Reinertsen, M.D.
Fred A. Rice, M.D.
Julie Rice, N.P.
Theresa A. Ryan, M.D.
William F. Schoenwetter, M.D.
Alvin L. Schultz, M.D.
Norman A. Sterrie, M.D.
James G. Stolhanske
William F. Telleen
James V. Toscano
Gerald P. Utley
Donald G. Velleck, M.D.
Loren N. Vorlicky, M.D.
Mary Lee Webber
Steve Wetzell
Asher A. White, Jr., M.D.
Leonard G. Wilson, Ph.D.

PREFACE

Over the last seventy-five years, health care has undergone the most profound changes in all of recorded history. This period of momentous change parallels the history of Park Nicollet, which has lived through, been part of, and in some major ways contributed to these changes. On the occasion of the seventy-fifth anniversary of Park Nicollet, we are pleased to publish this volume, documenting the development of one of the foremost multispecialty group clinics in the United States today.

Rather than the typical "coffee table" oversized picture book, a monument to past achievement, we have endeavored to produce a readable history that provides an understanding of the current clinic and its development and that serves as a preface to our future.

This work has been a labor of love for the Institute for Research and Education, formerly the Park Nicollet Medical Foundation, and we are most pleased and gratified by its publication.

This book follows the work of many others; significant among them are S. Marx White, Robert Newell, Roger Asplin, William Costello, Alex Barno, Bud Green, and Mark Peacock. We are most indebted to Jim Hare, who spent hundreds of hours interviewing our colleagues and reading histories, minutes, newspapers, newsletters, correspondence, personal memoirs, and related material to bring about this final effort. We are also grateful to Karol Carstensen, Gail Devery, and Judy Peacock for the wonderful editing and depth of publishing experience that made this book possible.

Finally, we want to thank the founders of the Nicollet Clinic and the St. Louis Park Medical Center for their vision in creating a multispecialty group practice that is based on the values of excellent patient care, continuing research and education, and service to patients and community. Park Nicollet is an extraordinary center for health care, research, and education of which we can all be proud. It is a privilege to work in an environment based on these values, and it is our responsibility to uphold them as we continue to serve the needs of our patients and the community.

A. Stuart Hanson, M.D.
President and Chief Executive Officer

James V. Toscano
Executive Vice President

PART ONE

THE NICOLLET CLINIC

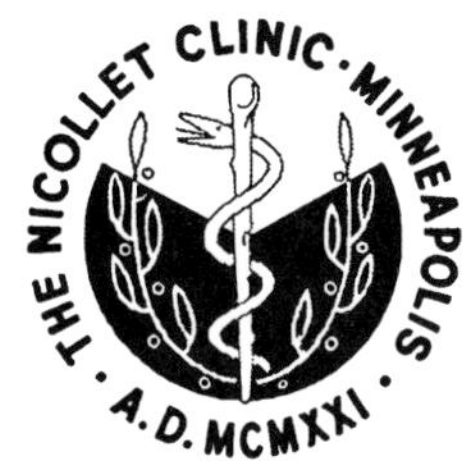

1

INVENTING GROUP PRACTICE

THE FOUNDING OF THE NICOLLET CLINIC

In the early spring of 1919, the University of Minnesota Medical School was struggling to return to normal as the doctors assigned to Base Hospital 26 returned home from France. The hospital had been organized by the medical school in 1917 at the request of the War Department. It included some "300 doctors, nurses, pharmacists, technicians, and maintenance people" recruited from the staffs of the University of Minnesota and Mayo Clinic and from the community.[1] The hospital's commissioned medical officers, including one S. Marx White, had organized it by specialty to best utilize the talents of the physician staff. This method of organizing medical services came naturally to the physician-academics of Minnesota and served them well during their seven-month tour of duty in France.

As any veteran will acknowledge, the unity of purpose experienced by a company of soldiers is not easily forgotten. So it was natural for two veteran physicians of Base Hospital 26, Gilbert Thomas and Angus Morrison, to share tales in December 1919 while traveling by train to the annual meeting of the Southern Minnesota Medical Association in Mankato. As the snow-covered fields and farms drifted by, their reminiscences turned to a spirited discussion of the possibility of creating a group of medical specialists made up of members of Base Hospital 26.

Thomas, then thirty-five and an assistant professor of urology at the University of Minnesota, was not one to let a good idea slip away. His friend Angus Morrison, a year older and an assistant professor in the medical school's neurology department, was also attracted to the idea, and the two resolved to pursue the project among their colleagues and fellow war veterans.

ASSEMBLING THE GROUP

Charles Reed was the first to be approached. Ten years older with a busy orthopedics practice in downtown Minneapolis, Reed also held a staff appointment in orthopedic surgery at the university. Intrigued by the possibility of recreating the spirit of cooperative medicine he had experienced as a major at Base Hospital 26, Reed signed up without hesitation. Dr. Louis Baldwin was the next to come on board. As superintendent of the university's hospital, Baldwin had taken on the task of organizing the medical equipment for Base Hospital 26 and had then spent the remainder of the war years in Washington, D.C., directing personnel and administration in the Office of the Surgeon General. A natural selection as the group's administrator and business manager, Baldwin agreed to join the others for a conversation with their former leader, S. Marx White.

As White remembered their proposal in his autobiography, he "had been giving thought to the same idea, but had devised no way of procedure."[2] White had been teaching pathology and internal medicine at the university medical school for twenty-one years and would, in two years, be named chief of the Department of Medicine. He, too, signed onto the idea without reservations.

With the addition of White, the group forged ahead, refining the concept and seeking to include those men on the university staff who would bring "professional competence, a standing in the community, the ability to work in cooperation and experience as teachers" to the group. The planners decided they needed someone on whom to test their idea. The man they selected, "the piercing of whose armor would be a test of the quality of our ammunition," in White's words, and "whose acceptance of the plan would give the assurance to proceed," was the respected professor of obstetrics and gynecology, Jennings C. Litzenberg.

"Litz," as he was known to his friends, was no stranger to S. Marx White. They had, since 1908, shared private practice office space in the downtown Donaldson Building, and their families had shared an apartment in Vienna for several months in 1914 while the two of them studied the techniques of the renowned Austrian specialists at the Allgemeine Krankenhaus, then the largest hospital in the world.[3] So it was natural that White be nominated to approach Litzenberg with the idea of creating a new multispecialty clinic in Minneapolis.

As chief of the Department of Obstetrics and Gynecology at the university and president of the Hennepin County Medical Society, Litzenberg cast a long shadow in the Minnesota medical community. Litzenberg "had a very valuable approach," White recorded in his memoirs, "and could easily think of more objections than I could conjure in a week." As a man at the top of his field, Litzenberg was used to coming to his own conclusions and "had to be approached from the side."[4] And so it was that White began to drop by the Litzenberg residence on Sunday afternoons for a series of "neighborly chats in front of his fireplace" with his strong-willed friend and colleague.[5] Each time, the conversation would turn to the need for a well-organized clinic in Minneapolis until, one day as White was taking his leave, Litzenberg said to him, "That clinic idea appeals to me. Why don't you see if anyone else would be interested?" White wasted no time contacting the rest of the group with the news.[6]

The first recorded meetings of the group occurred early in 1920 and included Drs. Thomas, Morrison, Reed, White, Litzenberg, and Baldwin. Each of the members put $100 into an account under Baldwin's care to cover organizing expenses, legal fees, and the like. By July 1920, three more members were added to the group. William R. Murray was chief of the Department of Ophthalmology, Otolaryngology, and Rhinology at the university and a member of the Minnesota Academy of Ophthalmology. At the time the group was forming, Murray was associated with the Children's Clinic at Abbott Hospital, and he urged the group to exclude pediatrics from the clinic as a condition of his joining. This was quickly accepted with an added commitment that it was the group's "intention and desire . . . to cooperate with the Minneapolis Children's Clinic."[7]

The next physician to join was Arthur C. Strachauer, chief of the university's Department of Surgery. Strachauer was known by his students as a colorful and interesting lecturer, and by his colleagues as a versatile and skillful surgeon. His handsome and commanding presence made him an ideal "front man" for the clinic.

John P. Schneider, an associate professor of internal medicine at the university, was next to be offered membership in the group. He accepted the invitation of his colleagues in June 1920 and was promptly put to work with Thomas to design a laboratory to serve the new clinic. In August, the group agreed to include a tenth member, James A. Johnson, Strachauer's deputy in the university's surgery department.

With their roster of senior partners complete, the details of hammering out an organizational philosophy and of creating a corporation dominated the twice weekly meetings, which continued through most of the summer of 1920. Though they were challenging the traditions of independence valued by a majority of their colleagues in medicine, the group was part of a widespread movement in the United States. Of 330 private medical groups identified in a 1940 study by the Public Health Service, 25 percent, or 82 of them had formed between 1919 and 1923. The report concluded that the experience of military service, "which accustomed them to cooperative, disciplined organization . . . probably contributed" to the formation of many of the medical groups during this period.[8]

IDEALS AND ORGANIZATION

The "year of companionship in France" with Base Hospital 26, as S. Marx White once wrote, "was one of the influences" that led to the formation of the Nicollet Clinic and its multispecialty approach.[9] But it was by no means the only factor. The Mayo Clinic, already a dominant force in Minnesota medicine, helped to blaze this path. William Mayo was a vocal advocate of medical group practice. As early as 1910, Mayo and his brother Charles were exhorting their colleagues to "develop medicine as a cooperative science: the clinician, the specialist, the laboratory workers, uniting for the good of the patient. . . . Individualism in medicine," they said, "can no longer exist."[11]

To be sure, the group practice of medicine as an ideal had not yet been accepted by a majority of physicians in 1920. The individual power granted by the growing arsenal of effective remedies and methods was heady indeed for the general practitioner. But in the more idealistic world of the established, practicing clinical professors who came together in Minneapolis at this time, the message preached by the Mayo brothers could be evaluated on its merit and was wholeheartedly embraced.

The first articles of incorporation of the group, written in October 1920, established that the "purpose of the corporation [would be] to enable its members to unite their efforts for the more effectual practice of medicine and surgery; [to own and operate] labs and hospitals for the care and treat-

"We had no desire to grow to the size of the Mayo Clinic. . . . We would cooperate fully with the University of Minnesota and the University Hospital. We did not propose to establish research laboratories, nor be particularly eager to join in new procedures such as were beginning at the University Medical School. Rather, in our situation, we would let developments and improvements occur as they were presented in our work. . . . Any additions to the staff would have to have unanimous approval. Our aim was the pursuit of excellence and it was believed that inept or undesirable members might thus be avoided. . . . Free consultation between departments was encouraged. We could thus learn one from the other." [10]

S. Marx White

ment of those in need . . . [and for] affording gratuitous ministrations to the indigent and distressed; [and] to afford instruction and opportunity for research."[12] This statement of purpose put the group squarely in the camp of the medical reformers of the day. Group practice was a way to bring the principles of modern industry to the private practice of medicine through specialization and organization.

This commitment to group practice was matched by an equally strong commitment to preserving the ideal of the doctor-patient relationship. In White's words, the group believed that "every patient is the particular charge of one physician and not of the clinic as a whole," and that physician, acting as a general practitioner, "is responsible for the integration of all the data."[13] The belief that private group practice could enhance the doctor-patient relationship was part of the bedrock faith of the founding group.

With a common understanding and commitment to the ideals of group practice established, the group turned to the gritty details of organizing and running a medical clinic.

FINANCIAL RELATIONSHIP

Throughout the summer of 1920, the group hammered out the details of an agreement that would govern the financial relationship between the individual physicians and the group as a whole. The compromise that was struck reflected the general sentiment that each of the partners should participate equally in whatever income was generated. This egalitarian tendency had to be balanced against the financial chasm that separated the high- and low-earning partners. John Schneider, who had spent the war years building his private internal medicine practice, reported a private practice income of $36,000, almost seven times the $5,500 declared by Morrison and Reed. Although little of the discussion is recorded, the bylaws of the corporation, approved in October 1920, clearly established a time line and distribution formula by which equal compensation, regardless of specialty, would be achieved.

It was, the group agreed, the "duty of every member of the corporation to devote his entire working time to the business and affairs of the corporation." Reflecting their desire to retain close ties to the university, the definition of "work" included time spent at the university "to the use and benefit of the corporation." All fees would go to the corporation where net income would be redistributed as salaries based on the formula established in the bylaws. Paid vacation time was set at a very liberal "not to exceed two months," at least part of which was to be used for attending professional meetings and for additional training. Resignation from the group would require six-months' notice. Members would be entitled to a proportionate share of the property of the corporation upon resignation or death. With the outline of a financial agreement in place, each of the members agreed to put up $4,200 as a loan to the corporation to cover operating expenses and start-up costs.

FACILITIES AND STAFFING

As 1920 was drawing to a close, the group's first employee, Mrs. F. L. Fridley, was hired to assist Dr. Baldwin at the excellent salary of $3,000 per year. Baldwin, having shouldered administrative responsibilities for the group, had located 13,000 square feet of second-floor office space in a new building at the corner of 10th Street and Nicollet Avenue in downtown Minneapolis. A ten-year lease with the Intercity Realty and Loan Company was drafted and signed. Proposed floor plans were examined, discussed, and revised many times. The lease, with a first-year cost of $24,350, was assumed by the new corporation in October 1920.

With an executive committee consisting of William Murray, S. Marx White, and J. C. Litzenberg, and functional committees to help him, Baldwin directed the procurement of office furnishings, laboratory equipment, and X-ray equipment. A budget of $7,700 was approved for the laboratory and the X-ray equipment, with an additional $4,500 for the purchase of an electrocardiograph.

Baldwin next turned his attention to staffing. The group had identified several younger physicians, most from the university, whom they wished to bring on board as "professional associates." One of the first of these associates contacted by Baldwin, at the request of S. Marx White, was the young internist Olga S. Hansen. A former student and long-time friend of White's, and an expert in the new field of electrocardiography, Hansen would remain with the Nicollet Clinic for over fifty years.

Other associates were contacted and hired into the group. James B. Carey, an internist, was brought in to work with Dr. Schneider. F. H. K. Schaaf, another internist, joined Dr. White. Obstetricians William Condit and Manley H. Haynes joined Litzenberg's department. In all, five associate physicians were members of the group in 1921.

Hoping to provide a well-rounded clinic, the founding group decided to bring in a dentist and to establish a pharmacy. Everett E. MacGibbon, an associate professor at the University of Minnesota and a consultant in oral surgery with Base Hospital 26, was offered and accepted the dental position. The James A. Malerich Pharmacy agreed to operate a pharmacy in space leased by the clinic on the first floor. The pharmacy opened with the clinic and continued, through several name changes, to serve patients and the public at that location for the next forty years.

Baldwin and the Executive Committee continued to recruit professional and office staff. By opening day, nine office and maintenance staff and nine "office assistants" (nurses) had been hired to support the professional staff of physicians and associates.

NAMING THE GROUP

What's in a name? For the founders the answer to this question was "very much indeed." The ideal name would avoid using any of the names of the organizers. It would not unduly "antagonize our friends in the medical community" and it should favor no specialty or group within the clinic.[14]

The group at first settled on "The Minneapolis Group Clinic, Inc.," but it was soon discarded. Two more names, "Medical and Surgical Clinic of Minneapolis, Inc.," adopted on the day the group signed its lease at 10th and Nicollet, and "The Minnesota Clinic of Minneapolis, Inc.," were tried before the group settled on a suggestion made by Charles Reed, "The Nicollet Clinic of Minneapolis, Inc."[15] Fourth choice though it was, the name served the clinic well, evoking as it did the location of the clinic on Minneapolis' best shopping street and the romantic image of Jean Nicholas Nicollet, one of the region's early explorers.

A QUIET OPENING

As the group got closer to opening day, news of their activities began to circulate and piqued the interest of the local newspapers. But in the medical profession of 1920, publicity was something to be absolutely avoided if possible. At the time, professional ethics prohibited any promotion of a physician's services. Creating a cooperative group was itself near the edge of acceptable behavior, and the group's activities had already generated "considerable criticism and some enmity" within professional circles.[16] Many physicians were suspicious and uncertain of the effect a group clinic might have on their individual practices. If allowed to grow, this uncertainty could threaten the new multispecialty practice, which required referrals from many individual

FOUNDERS OF THE NICOLLET CLINIC JANUARY 25, 1921

Louis B. Baldwin,
Business Administration
James A. Johnson,
Surgery
Jennings C. Litzenberg,
Obstetrics/Gynecology
Angus W. Morrison,
Neuropsychiatry
William R. Murray,
Eye, Ear, Nose, Throat
Charles A. Reed,
Orthopedics
John P. Schneider,
Internal Medicine
Arthur C. Strachauer,
Surgery
Gilbert J. Thomas,
Urology
S. (Solon) Marx White,
Internal Medicine

ASSOCIATES

James B. Carey,
Internal Medicine
William H. Condit,
Obstetrics/Gynecology
Olga S. Hansen,
Internal Medicine
Manley H. Haynes,
Obstetrics/Gynecology
Everett E. MacGibbon,
Dentistry
F. H. K. Schaaf,
Internal Medicine

practitioners. Prominent press coverage, the group was reasonably certain, would unnecessarily add fuel to the fires of opposition in the medical fraternity.

The group called on its two most prominent members, S. Marx White and J. C. Litzenberg, to manage the public announcement of incorporation and the opening of the clinic. Through "quick and positive action," the exact nature of which was not recorded, the "publicity committee" managed to suppress "projects for popular write-ups."[17] The group did, however, send announcements of their opening and address changes to colleagues in the medical profession in Minneapolis and St. Paul and to patients of the members.

The Nicollet Clinic opened without fanfare on January 25, 1921, a full-fledged multispecialty group, complete with a pharmacy, a dentist, a diagnostic laboratory, and X-ray facilities. The ideas, ideals, and patient organizing of the ten founders had borne fruit.

2

IDEALISTS MEET REALITY

THE NICOLLET CLINIC 1921 TO 1934

As the postwar recession closed in on the Twin Cities in 1921, social tensions increased, most dramatically evidenced by the violent strikes at the South St. Paul stockyards. The government, meanwhile, was having difficulty enforcing the prohibition against alcohol consumption. Lawlessness and disrespect were being distilled as surely as home brew. Minneapolis, already in the midst of a transformation from a lumber and milling town to a financial and trading service center, was becoming a center of bootlegger activity. The economic hardship in the rural Midwest was causing a migration into the region's cities, and Minneapolis itself became something of a boomtown.

From the physician's perspective these were tremendously exciting times. The entire character of medicine was changing. Scientific knowledge of the human organism—its functions, malfunctions, and diseases—was expanding exponentially. Advances in laboratory diagnostic and surgical techniques were vastly improving the physician's ability to effect the outcome of disease in the individual. Pretending to know the full spectrum of the physician's craft was no longer possible, and specialty associations were organizing rapidly and contesting for authority over various medical territories. The founders of the Nicollet Clinic contributed many hours to the efforts of their specialty organizations.

ECONOMIC REALITIES

The more immediate concern toward the end of 1921, however, was the financial survival of the group. The contracting economy, the group's failure to collect almost one-third of the accounts billed, and an overestimation of the first year's bookings left the clinic with far less income than had been expected. A mere $75,000 was distributed to the ten members of the corporation at the end of their first year—over $100,000 less than had been projected in January.

As bad as the financial report was in 1921, it wasn't bad enough to shake the group's faith in their project. They were determined to keep charges as low as possible and to maintain their commitment to group practice. Various efforts to improve the finances of the group were tried in 1922, but by November of that year the members realized that their initial loan of operating capital to the clinic was unlikely to be repaid. The group members agreed to gift their $4,200 investments to the clinic. This must have been a painful decision on the part of the younger members in particular, as the amount represented almost a year's salary for some. Additional loans representing the cash value of the equipment each member had brought into the practice were to be paid off as funds became available.

To more effectively manage collections and billing, Alfred G. Stasel, a young accountant and attorney who had prepared the group's first annual financial report, was hired in October 1922 on a part-time basis. Stasel, described as "hard-boiled in money matters,"[18] quickly gained the confidence of the physicians.

Alfred Stasel believed that every patient would pay for medical services, provided the fee was within the realm of his or her ability to pay. Consequently, the clinic developed a sliding-fee system, a typical practice of turn-of-the-century physicians. Each patient's account was given a symbol corresponding to one of eight categories of net worth and annual income, from "charity" with no income to "AAA" with an income of over $15,000. At the conclusion of the case, the business office totaled the fee on the standard fee schedule and automatically adjusted it to the economic circumstances of the patient. A physical exam with a standard fee of $75 would thus cost a patient anywhere from $30 to $90 depending on the patient's income. The physician, Stasel reported to his colleagues at the Association of Clinic Managers, "is left free to render his services without any question as to whether it is a bank president or the janitor in the bank."[19] The sliding-fee schedule was phased out in 1948.

With Stasel's constant attention and business expertise, collections soon began to gain on bookings. However, despite a steady and substantial growth in revenues and income, the disappointing shortfall between promised and actual salaries continued. This tended to squeeze those near the bottom of the distribution schedule beyond tolerance. Gilbert Thomas, one of the younger doctors, forced the issue in 1924 when he resigned, citing financial hardship. Thomas happily withdrew his resignation after the group agreed to salary guarantees for himself and James Johnson.

Reviewing 1924 as outgoing president, internist John Schneider reported the net worth of the corporation had risen to $177,000. This was a "very dependable worth" in his view, given that each member was assured upon withdrawal or death at least 80 to 85 percent cash realization of the assets. Schneider compared this with the 35 to 40 percent typically realized by an individual physician on ceasing practice. "This factor is of such great importance," he said, "that it cannot be too frequently emphasized in view of the uncertainty of life."[20]

In his annual address, Schneider also expressed his long-held opposition to the salary equalization formula. "Our idealistic dream of ultimate equality is, I am sure, a proven dream by this, our fourth birthday," he said. "Men's professional ability, energy, vision and salesmanship differ as widely as their ability to direct and conserve their own earnings." The loss of a large book of minutes prevents knowing exactly when the ideal of an equal partnership was finally given up. It remains a fact, however, that during the first few years, with incomes far below that projected in 1920, the partnership income was distributed much more equally than it might have been.

Schneider ended his summary of 1924 on a cautiously optimistic note. "With year by year a better understanding of the nature of group practice; with the gradual elimination of some of our vestigial habits of isolated thought and action . . . ; with more consultation . . . due patience and humanity, we will, I am certain, as the years unroll, find ourselves in smooth water, with a ship far more stable than the usual professional vessel in the evening of our lives."[21]

PROFESSIONAL OPPOSITION

Collecting on their accounts was not the only challenge the group faced in the early years. As part of a new movement creating multispecialty group medicine, they faced cloaked hostility from the larger medical profession, which insisted that only the independent general practitioner could guarantee a satisfactory doctor-patient relationship. Shortly after the clinic opened in 1921, an editorial in the *Journal of the American Medical Association* wondered if group practice would lead to the elimination of the general practitioner. "Does [group practice] mean that the family physician is being replaced by a corporation?" asked the editorial. Calling forth the established medical profession's greatest fear, the editorial went on to ask, "How will the layman view it? Will he not prefer state medicine?"[22]

The American Medical Association opposed the corporate practice of medicine more explicitly. In 1929 the Judicial Council of the association decreed that "the practice of medicine by corporations . . . is detrimental to the best interest of scientific medicine and of the people themselves."[23] The Minnesota State Medical Association, the state affiliate, adopted this position and worked strenuously to outlaw the practice of medicine by corporations. Technically, this applied to the Nicollet Clinic, as it was organized as a corporation. However, the leadership of the state affiliate was not interested in challenging the clinic on this point, as evidenced by the fact that Jennings Litzenberg was elected to a three-year term as a state representative to the medical association's national House of Delegates in 1928.[24]

Back in Minneapolis, opposition to group practice in general and the Nicollet Clinic in particular was muted by the prominence of the group's members as teachers and practitioners and by the influence of the Mayo Clinic. Although the Nicollet Clinic founders never publicly recorded the opposition they faced, it remains a distinct memory of those who knew the group privately. Clinton Morrison, Dr. Angus Morrison's son, remembers the formation of the Nicollet Clinic causing "an uproar in the medical profession." Dr. Asher White, son of S. Marx White, who joined his father in the Nicollet Clinic in 1933, credited the "opposition of the local physicians outside the clinic who opposed the idea of physicians banding together" with a successful effort to strip hospital privileges from clinic doctors.[25]

This particular story involved the decision by the medical staff of Abbott Hospital to bar Nicollet Clinic physicians from its staff—a particularly galling decision, as Abbott was regarded as the premier hospital in Minneapolis. It was the hospital of choice for many of the wealthier clients of the clinic and the hospital to which James Johnson had advocated concentrating all surgery in 1921.[26]

PURCHASING EITEL HOSPITAL

It had long been apparent that significant time and cost savings might be accomplished by consolidating the doctors' hospital work and integrating it with their work at the clinic. Discussion of how this might be accomplished had been going on since the first year of operation. Group members had visited private clinic/hospitals in Chicago and Cleveland to gather ideas. Ruling out building their own hospital, the group had decided by the mid-1920s to look for an opportunity to purchase an existing hospital.[27] The experience of being "thrown out" of Abbott added urgency to the decision to establish hospital access for the entire clinic staff in a single, well-run facility.

The clinic and Eitel Hospital had an amicable relationship, which began in 1922 when the group accepted hospital privileges there. Founded in 1914 by Dr. George G. Eitel, a prominent Minneapolis surgeon, and his wife, Jeanette, a nurse and hospital administrator,[28] the hospital was, according to the *Journal Lancet* in 1920, a model of cost-conscious, high-quality service.[29] Overlooking Loring Park at 14th and Willow streets, the 130-bed hospital was located only eight blocks from the offices of the Nicollet Clinic.

Soon after her husband died in the early spring of 1928, Jeanette Eitel approached the clinic about purchasing Eitel Hospital. Negotiations continued through the winter and by the spring of 1929 an acceptable agreement was reached. The $185,000 sale price was financed with a $125,000 mortgage from the First Minneapolis Trust Co., with the balance raised from seventeen members of the Nicollet Clinic—including Alfred G. Stasel, now the group's full-time business administrator.[30] The land itself was retained by Mrs. Eitel, with a one-hundred-year ground lease granted to the Nicollet Clinic beginning on April 1, 1929. The lease gave the clinic a five-year option to purchase the land for an additional $183,333. Consistent with the group's desire to create an integrated clinic/hospital, the land lease also contained a clause specifying that a new building worth at least $150,000 would be built on the property within five years, with a $50,000 penalty for failure to build within ten years.[31]

A new corporation, Nicollet Hospitals, Inc., was chartered in Delaware to hold and operate the hospital. Although the hospital corporation was a separate entity, the Nicollet Clinic was given the right to appoint ten of the fifteen board members. The hospital's existing staff of medical professionals was retained, as was the medical staff organization, including all physicians whether or not they were on the clinic staff.[32] Alfred Stasel assumed the job of hospital administrator. The group had now solved the question of hospital access and control, but the realization of any financial benefit to the clinic of this early attempt at integration would have to wait. Within the year the stock market had collapsed, and the Great Depression was officially underway.

THE DEPRESSION YEARS

Just as it tested the strength of the nation, the Great Depression provided the greatest test yet of the vision and commitment of the founders of the Nicollet Clinic. Physicians across the country saw their incomes fall by 50 percent, as fewer and fewer people sought care. Collection of accounts fell as the people who did come in shuffled the doctor's bill to the bottom of a growing pile—to be paid last, if ever.[33] By one estimate, 42 percent of private practice groups failed to survive the 1930s.[34]

The financial situation at the Nicollet Clinic was no exception. Bookings fell from a high in 1928 of $322,888 to only $141,005 in 1933.[35] Admissions to Eitel Hospital fell by 50 percent. As their practice shrank, the physicians

As the clinic grew during the 1920s, it had become a custom for Alfred Stasel to schedule the annual meeting at the Minneapolis Club. His successor, Robert Newell, recalls a founder's story of how "he could always tell when the financial report was going to be bad . . . the cocktail hour would run long and after dinner, drinks would be served. "During the Depression years," the founders would say, "the cocktail and dinner part of the program got very long indeed."

found creative, and not so creative, ways to fill their days. The ardent golfers spent more time on the links. On slow days, those that weren't out playing golf set up a bridge table in the Eye, Ear, Nose, and Throat waiting room. The few patients who would appear barely interrupted the game.[36]

This "enforced leisure" was the subject S. Marx White took up in a 1933 article in the *Bulletin of the Hennepin County Medical Society*. Ever the teacher, White suggested that his fellow underemployed doctors visit the University of Minnesota. Its leaders, he wrote, were "surprisingly hospitable to new ideas and workers" and ready to "show us the places in which something may be added" to the present body of medical knowledge. "Now that an enforced leisure has proved to us we can survive on the product of fewer hours labor," he went on, "may we not learn to use that leisure for the common good and develop a finer, truer culture?" [37]

UNIVERSITY LEADERSHIP

Many of White's colleagues were already active on campus. Indeed, as professors and former department heads at the University Medical School, the founders of the Nicollet Clinic maintained their close ties to the university.

Arthur Strachauer

Surgeon Arthur Strachauer provides a good example of the solid record of achievement and commitment to the university established by the founders during the clinic's first twenty years. Strachauer, the university's chief of surgery from 1919 to 1925, is credited by medical historian Leonard Wilson with setting medical student Owen S. Wangensteen on the path to a surgical specialty. Wangensteen, living up to the expectations of his mentor, became chief of surgery in 1930, and subsequently led the University of Minnesota to the top of surgical research and instruction.[38]

Under Strachauer's leadership the Nicollet Clinic, in cooperation with the university's graduate program, established a fellowship in surgery in 1922. The department took on two additional surgical assistants that year, and a steady parade of young surgeons came to work with Strachauer and James Johnson in the clinic. Thomas J. Kinsella, the first such assistant, later became a leading thoracic surgeon, completing the first successful total extirpation of a lung for carcinoma in Minnesota in 1937.[39]

Louis Baldwin

Louis Baldwin, who had kept his position as superintendent of the university's hospital after the opening of the Nicollet Clinic, was in the thick of the struggle to find the resources to build an adequate medical school facility. Under his direction, the Todd and Christian buildings were added to the university hospital in 1926, bringing the total number of beds to over three hundred.[40]

Jennings C. Litzenberg

Jennings Litzenberg never really left the university. Appointed to head the new combined department of obstetrics and gynecology in 1913, Litzenberg continued in that capacity until his retirement in 1938. His clinical observations in 1922 of the relationship between hypothyroidism and sterility were reported in a series of journal articles beginning in 1926. He was the discoverer of the "Litzenberg embryo," the youngest embryo identified at the time. The Kansas Obstetrical and Gynecological Society called him the "dean of American obstetrics."[41] Litzenberg's natural leadership and his many contributions were further recognized when he was elected president of

Widowed at the peak of his career in 1927, Litzenberg married Olga Hansen in 1934, much to the delight of the clinic grapevine. Their home on East River Road became a frequent gathering place for all manner of medical meetings, student groups, and university football booster parties.

the American Association of Obstetricians, Gynecologists and Abdominal Surgeons.

Litzenberg also was an outspoken proponent of the need to reduce the maternal death rate in the state and the nation. When he accepted the chair of obstetrics and gynecology at the university in 1913, the maternal mortality rate in Minnesota was 7 per 1,000 births. Under the guidance of Litzenberg, Minnesota achieved the lowest maternal death rate in the country in 1927 and, by 1947, Minnesota had a record of .6 maternal deaths per 1,000 births, the lowest ever recorded.[42]

Olga Hansen

Olga Hansen's skill with the electrocardiograph won her an appointment to head the cardiac clinic at the university hospital in 1917, a post she held until 1927. Hansen was also interested in diabetes and quickly grasped the importance of insulin, isolated for the first time in 1922 by Dr. Frederick Banting and Charles Best. She was the first physician in Minneapolis to treat a private patient with the new drug.[43] Active in the Hennepin County Medical Society, Hansen served as the associate editor of the Bulletin from its first issue in 1929 until 1940 and as a member of the society's executive committee from 1931 to 1934.

S. Marx White

Like his good friend Jennings Litzenberg, S. Marx White never really left the university. He had taught pathology and internal medicine since 1898 and had been a full professor of internal medicine since 1915. When the chief of medicine, Leonard Rowntree, left unexpectedly for the Mayo Foundation in 1920, White assumed leadership of the department. White remained head of the department until 1925 and continued on as an active clinical professor until 1942. In 1931, White became president of the American College of Physicians. During a period when the state legislature seemed uninterested in granting money to the university's medical school, part-time faculty leaders like White and Litzenberg helped to raise private funds to improve and maintain the school's facilities.

In the August 1960 issue of the Journal Lancet, *Dr. Catherine Corson West noted that Olga Hansen served as a role model for many young women. West first met Hansen at the Nicollet Clinic in 1922 while working as a switchboard operator.*

Others

Most of the others in the group continued to maintain a connection to the university. William Condit, for instance, taught obstetrics and gynecology at the university from 1914 until 1938. Gilbert Thomas taught urology as an associate clinical professor for many years and also became president of the American Urologic Society in 1937. Another founder, James Johnson, began as an instructor in the department of surgery and was named clinical professor in 1941. Charles Reed taught orthopedic surgery at the university for thirty years and contributed significantly to knowledge of tuberculosis of the bones and joints.

THE CLINIC MATURES

As the clinic's fifteenth anniversary approached in 1936, the group could look back on a solid record of achievement and growth through the toughest of times. Tested by the Depression and by skeptics in their own profession, the group had maintained their commitment to group practice and continued to offer a full range of medical services despite the loss of some of the founding members.

Louis Baldwin was the first of the original members to leave the corporation. His multiple roles as administrator of the Nicollet Clinic, superintendent of the university hospital, and organizer of the new Miller Hospital in St. Paul had aggravated his hypertension. Wishing to lighten

Tragedy struck the clinic in December 1926, when Dr. William Murray, performing a routine mastoid operation, pricked his finger. The Minneapolis Daily Star, *under the banner headline proclaiming him a "Martyr to His Profession," recounted the harrowing story: "Although the poison was working up through his hand, Dr. Murray coolly continued the operation, which he performed successfully. Then he cauterized the wound and anticipated he would throw off the infection. By the next morning his entire left arm was affected and he was removed to the hospital. Murray died after several transfusions and the amputation of his left arm failed to check the ravages of the deadly infection."* [45]

his workload, he resigned from the clinic in 1924. With regrets the group accepted his resignation, acknowledging the need for his services by the University of Minnesota.[44]

Arthur Strachauer was the next of the founders to leave the group. With the Chase Cancer Center launched and his tour as caretaker of the university's surgery department completed, and perhaps feeling ready to devote more time to his interests in music and the outdoors, Strachauer resigned from the Nicollet Clinic in 1931 to accept the title of Chief Surgeon of the Soo Line Railroad. Angus Morrison also left the group in 1931, giving up the practice of medicine to devote more time to his family's many and substantial financial interests.

In 1932, after many years as salaried physicians, James Carey, William Condit, Olga Hansen, and Hugo Altnow, an internist who had joined the group in 1925, were invited to become members of the corporation. With the addition of several physicians and in spite of the hardships imposed on the community by the Great Depression, the clinic continued to offer services in each of the major specialties. When Minneapolis hit bottom in 1933, the clinic employed seventeen physicians and three dentists in nine specialty divisions: ophthalmology, urology, surgery, bone surgery, dentistry, neurology, internal medicine, obstetrics, and pediatrics. The newest division, pediatrics, was created in September 1933 by Dr. Stuart L. Arey.

Their individual achievements notwithstanding, the foundation of the group's success rested on the joy the members found in their work and in each other. Walter Haven, a dentist who was employed by the group in 1923 and who later rejoined as a physician, remembers the group dynamic as one "with no friction or antagonisms. There were wonderful discussions every Friday at their luncheons."[46] Hints of the good humor of this group are scattered throughout issues of the *Bulletin of the Hennepin County Medical Society* during this period.

A mimeographed poster announcing the "Nicollet Clinic

Circus" is perhaps the best surviving example of the humor and joy in work that lie hidden just below the surface of the meeting minutes and official histories. The summer clinic picnic at the Morrison home on Lake Minnetonka had become a tradition by 1925. "Coming!! Coming!! Coming!!" the poster reads. "One Day Only - The Famous, Factitious, Fibricient, Fribillating Nicollet Clinic Circus." The attractions at this circus? A partial list includes "Morrisini's Troupe of Pachycephalic Pachyderms"; "Baldy - The Strong Man, See Him Hold His Temper"; "Marxo - The Wild Man Tears Their Hearts Out and Eats 'Em Alive"; "Staselisti - In His Justly Famous Balancing Act"; and "Our Litz as Slivers the Clown." These physicians were people who liked words and each other.

3

REBUILDING FOR GROWTH

THE NICOLLET CLINIC 1935 TO 1956

"During the polio epidemics in the early 1950s, there was grave concern about transporting patients, so we would go out to their hospitals and see the patients and accompany them back to the city in the ambulance if necessary. We developed a tremendous loyalty in those towns by being willing to come out when they really needed us."

Arnold Anderson, M.D.

The late 1930s were heady times for medicine in the United States. The medical schools here had overtaken their European counterparts as the leading centers of medical innovation and research. The sulfanilamide compounds, introduced at Johns Hopkins in 1936, had launched the modern era of antibacterial chemotherapies. Public health efforts, based on better science and sanitation, were becoming increasingly effective. The campaign against tuberculosis, for example, was making slow progress against this dreaded killer, and the maternal health movement had dramatically reduced maternal death rates.

The sense of medical accomplishment was tempered by the daily reality of untreatable scourges such as polio, smallpox, and meningitis. Pediatrician Northrop Beach, who joined the Nicollet Clinic in 1943, remembers the "terrible ravages of things like meningitis" that were a daily reality on the hospital wards of the early 1940s before penicillin became widely available. The polio epidemics continued through the 1940s until the Salk and Sabin vaccines were introduced. "We spent August just worrying ourselves sick in the forties," is the way Beach described the anxiety parents and physicians felt as the yearly polio epidemic peaked through the late summer months.

Against this background the Nicollet Clinic strived to

rebuild from the economic devastation of the Great Depression. By 1936, its fifteenth anniversary, the clinic could see an end to the long struggle. Bookings were slowly increasing, although still only half the number recorded in 1928.

Five members of the founding group—S. Marx White, Jennings Litzenberg, Gilbert Thomas, Charles Reed, and James Johnson—still saw patients every day at the clinic. Several of the physicians were nearing retirement age, though most had no intention of retiring at age sixty-five. Younger associates and new partners were ready and anxious to assume leadership roles and found working with these eminent, but elderly, men at times "a little frustrating," according to Northrop Beach.

REORGANIZATION

Partly in response to the need to make room for the next generation, the clinic moved in 1935 to change its organizational structure. After fourteen years of operation as a for-profit corporation, in which the founders and a few others held the increasingly valuable shares, the clinic decided to reorganize as a partnership, called simply "The Nicollet Clinic." The existing corporation, The Nicollet Clinic of Minneapolis, Inc., was retained to hold title to the facilities and manage the business of the group.

In addition to providing a convenient way to broaden the ownership group, the change from a corporation to a partnership eliminated any appearance that the Nicollet Clinic may have been practicing "corporate" medicine, an issue of great interest to the state and national medical organizations at the time. The change also had the effect of allowing the members of the partnership to escape the new Social Security tax, the centerpiece of the New Deal and the very idea of which repulsed the more staunchly Republican members of the clinic.

With the changes completed by late 1937, the Nicollet Clinic was ready to "adopt a policy of Clinic growth, the taking in of younger men, for succession and perpetuation, for replacement or accession, [and] if the need arises the taking on of men with established practices."[47]

"Corporate medicine" is shorthand for the prohibition most states had enacted by the 1930s against corporations practicing medicine. An individual physician could be granted a license to practice medicine, but a corporation could not. Early interpretations of the law also effectively prohibited physicians from forming professional corporations, as lawyers were able to do. However, the Nicollet Clinic was organized before the Minnesota Basic Sciences Act, *passed in 1927, which set basic standards for the medical profession, established the state licensing board, and prohibited corporate medicine.*

WORLD WAR II INTERVENES

With the entry of the United States into World War II in 1941, however, the clinic's plans to take on new physicians were put on indefinite hold, as were the private plans of most Americans. Most of the younger physicians within the clinic—including internists Asher A. White and Gordon G. Bowers, obstetrician Raymond F. Cochrane, and surgeon Wallace I. Nelson—left for military duty. Their absence delayed the transfer of leadership to the next generation and the growth of the clinic.

With so many of the city's young physicians in the armed services, there was little chance of even temporarily replacing those called up. With a short staff and the return of prosperity, things got very busy at the Nicollet Avenue office for the staff that remained. In 1945, only eleven physicians handled 17 percent more patients than fourteen physicians had seen two years earlier.

THE HEALTH CARE DEBATE

Beginning in the 1930s and continuing into the 1940s, a war of words was occurring on the home front. At issue were the mechanisms and manner in which the achievements of medical science would be made available to all Americans. Progress in medicine had, by the time of the Great Depression, become synonymous with increasing costs—

costs often beyond the ability of families to pay out-of-pocket. As a result, labor, farm, and social justice organizations began advocating for a national system of health care insurance that would ensure access to medical care for all Americans. For a variety of reasons, the vast majority within the medical profession were passionately opposed to any government interference in the distribution or provision of medical care, as were others with a financial or ideological interest in preventing the socialization of health care.

The Nicollet Clinic physicians, as leaders of national stature, took a small, but significant, role in this debate. S. Marx White, who was serving as president of the American College of Physicians in 1932, used the occasion of his presidential address to urge the profession to shoulder the responsibility for ensuring access to medical care. "Bear in mind," he told his colleagues, "that only in the degree that we serve the public needs can we hope for, or receive, public approval. In England and Germany," he observed, "the imposition by legal enactment of certain intolerable and debasing conditions has been due in largest part to the refusal or failure of the medical profession in these countries to meet in adequate form the fundamental medical needs of the peoples involved."[48]

That same year the Roosevelt administration's Committee on the Cost of Medical Care strongly recommended providing comprehensive health care through multispecialty group practice as one step toward reducing costs and ensuring access, a position the physicians of the Nicollet Clinic supported in word and deed. But even this modest suggestion was opposed by much of the organized profession as an unacceptable interference in the private relationship between patients and their doctors. As the Depression rolled on, public pressure for a national solution to the health care worries families faced in every state culminated in the introduction of the Wagner National Health Care Bill in 1939. Once again, a Nicollet Clinic physician found it necessary to appeal for reasonable discourse. As president of the American Gynecological Society in 1941, Jennings Litzenberg told his assembled colleagues, "I cannot escape the belief that we will serve the public best by becoming more social-minded and less pugnacious. We cannot afford to have the impression grow that the profession is opposed to every social change."[49] But arguments for a reasoned debate fell by the wayside as a well-financed, ideologically driven campaign to discredit national health insurance got underway.

Pushed forward by the prospect of a national insurance plan, the medical profession turned to alternative structures to ensure broader access to medical services. In 1945, the Minnesota Medical Association worked for the passage of the Blue Shield law, which authorized groups of doctors to organize and operate not-for-profit medical plans. The association quickly gave its unanimous approval to the planning and implementation of the Minnesota Medical Service, the forerunner of Blue Shield of Minnesota. This new organization began offering a physician-sponsored, prepaid medical plan in November 1947. Similar physician-sponsored, locally administered prepayment plans were organized nationwide with the endorsement of the American Medical Association. The Nicollet Clinic voted to join the Blue Shield Plan in November 1948.[50]

The clinic was also experimenting with its own prepaid medical plan during this period. A contract to provide medical and hospital care to the members of the new Group Health Mutual, Inc., was finalized in 1941.[51] Group Health collected a monthly premium out of which fees were paid to the clinic for office care and to Eitel Hospital for regular hospital care. This program lasted until 1946, when a combination of inexperience with the actuarial data and postwar inflation pushed the costs of providing the service above what Group Health was willing to charge its membership. While a business failure in most respects, this prepaid medical plan provided the Nicollet Clinic with a steady stream of new patients, many of whom stayed with

Asher White wrote to congratulate the group on their silver anniversary from his post at Hanford, Washington. A member of the medical staff of the Manhattan Project, White praised the group's heritage of "group loyalty, high professional and ethical standards and never failing community of effort," which, he said, would "enable us to keep going far into the future." With the insight of a participant, he added, "These are the values which, in the new world of atomic energy, will be essential if the human race is to preserve itself on this planet."[52]

the clinic after the demise of the contract.

The national health care debate, which started with the New Deal and was pushed along heartily by President Harry Truman, collapsed with the election of Republican Dwight Eisenhower in 1952. The advocates of a national health insurance policy—having been repeatedly bashed as communist sympathizers—went into full retreat in the midst of the cold war hysteria of the 1950s.

POSTWAR CHANGES

The Nicollet Clinic had much to celebrate during its twenty-fifth anniversary dinner in January 1946. The nation was slowly demobilizing after the surrender of the Japanese only four months before. The clinic had posted a solid increase in bookings in spite of a short staff and was looking forward to the return of its veterans.

With the return of the World War II veterans, the clinic faced the problem of providing for the dignified transition to retirement of a significant proportion of its working physicians. As members of a partnership, none of the retiring physicians were then eligible for Social Security payments, nor had the clinic been able to establish a tax-deferred retirement plan such as those developed for employees of corporations. To smooth this transition, the clinic offered to repurchase each retiring physician's interest in the partnership over time, with the understanding that each could return as a salaried employee of the clinic. This arrangement had the additional advantage of qualifying the physician for the Social Security system. (Longtime partners Hugo Altnow, William Condit, and S. Marx White made this transition in 1952, all apparently converted to the idea of accepting a government pension.)

The next few years were a time of rapid growth and confidence. In 1947 the clinic accepted Melvin Baken Sr. into the partnership to replace retiring, long-time colleagues Jennings Litzenberg and William Condit. Baken, a prominent Minneapolis obstetrician, brought with him a large practice. His arrival helped shore up the obstetrics department, which was struggling to keep up with the first waves of the postwar baby boom. Patient visits to the clinic as a whole shot up by 65 percent between 1943 and 1947, driven by a quadrupling in the number of patients seen by the obstetrics department. Collections almost doubled during this period as well. In 1949, the group jumped at the chance to add Fred A. Rice, a Harvard Medical School graduate with residency training in internal medicine at the University of Chicago Hospital.

With the practice growing rapidly, the new leadership began to take a closer look at the practices of the business office. On the advice of business consultant Edwin L. Pearson, the partnership agreed to hire a new full-time manager to replace Alfred Stasel. Stasel at the time was managing both the clinic and Eitel Hospital as well as maintaining a busy schedule as a private hospital consultant. The older partners were less than enthusiastic about replacing the man who had "kept them in the black" through the Depression, but the new leadership had lost patience with Stasel's unaccountable style of management. After some negotiation, Stasel was eased out of the clinic in 1948, but retained his position as administrator of Eitel Hospital. On Pearson's recommendation, Robert Newell, a University of Minnesota Business School graduate and an experienced accountant, was hired in May 1948 to succeed Stasel.

CONTEMPLATING EXPANSION

As patient numbers grew rapidly after the war, the leased second-floor office on Nicollet Avenue, which had been

Talk of expanding the clinic had, by late 1953, created little but increased expectations. A minor staff revolt spilled into the inhouse newsletter, the Clinicscope. *Each of the first seven issues contained a "Why Don't We . . ." column that listed suggestions compiled from a suggestion box. "Why don't we build a new clinic?" ranked first in each issue. The column must have gotten under someone's skin. The eighth issue omitted it altogether, after the board asked that questions of policy be toned down or eliminated.*[54]

the group's location since 1921, became too small to house a modern multispecialty practice providing primary as well as specialty care. By 1948, the clinic was exploring options for expansion. A mezzanine in the existing building was renovated to create what Northrop Beach called "a wonderful and private space for pediatrics." The group considered purchasing the King Cole Hotel, which was on Willow Street near Loring Park, and transforming it into medical office space for the clinic and a convalescent home for Eitel Hospital. This idea was quickly dropped when the architect, Ellerbe and Associates, determined that the building could not be remodeled or redesigned into an effective medical clinic.[53] Another firm, Haarstick Lundgren and Associates, investigated adding a floor to the Nicollet Avenue office building, but this idea, too, was rejected.

Several other locations were investigated in early 1952, including a vacant site on Franklin and Blaisdell avenues. Marginally closer to the growing residential suburbs of south and west Minneapolis, the Blaisdell Avenue location was still close to Eitel Hospital and the University of Minnesota. Design drawings for a three-story clinic on Blaisdell Avenue were prepared and presented by Haarstick Lundgren in August 1952, and the board authorized the business office to proceed with negotiations to purchase the site. Negotiations continued unsuccessfully through the fall and winter, and were suspended when it became clear that the owner was willing to wait to get his price.

A MOVE TO THE SUBURBS?

With the rise of the automobile, people were moving farther and farther away from the downtown area. The near-south and western suburbs, in particular, were growing rapidly. For those patients who drove downtown in 1950 parking was tight and getting tighter. In a move that was perhaps twenty years ahead of its time, Northrop Beach opened a branch of the pediatrics department on Lyndale Avenue in Richfield, a suburb immediately south of Minneapolis. Run by pediatric nurse Ruth Erickson and staffed by Dr. Beach, the pioneering "satellite" clinic served patients from the Richfield, Bloomington, and Pilot Knob areas.[55]

The group was not interested, however, in following the pediatric department to the suburbs. Business Manager Robert Newell, still a fairly recent addition to the clinic staff, was well acquainted with the progress the new St. Louis Park Medical Center was making as a suburban, multispecialty clinic and was convinced that the Nicollet Clinic should move out of downtown to be closer to its patients. When Newell and John Dawson, an architect, suggested building a new clinic near Southdale Shopping Mall in Edina—where Dayton's was then building a new store—the board thought the two men had taken leave of their senses.[56] The partners were not about to abandon their long-standing ties to Eitel Hospital or their patients on the north side. They also were not willing to give up their ready access to the university or to the downtown medical community. At that time over 90 percent of the physicians practicing in Hennepin County still maintained offices within the city limits of Minneapolis.[57]

A VISION UNFULFILLED

Eitel Hospital stands out as an important influence on the development of the Nicollet Clinic. Purchased on the eve of the Great Depression, the hospital was the first step toward implementing the group's vision of an integrated hospital/clinic. Under the direction of Alfred Stasel and the Nicollet Clinic physicians, the hospital had survived the Depression with its reputation as a "high-class institution" intact. This was no small feat. Nationwide, over

Nicollet Hospitals, Inc., was originally chartered in Delaware to hold and operate Eitel Hospital. This arrangement did not satisfy the State of Minnesota, which considered the new corporation to be a for-profit taxable entity. When Hennepin County tried to collect property taxes on the hospital's property for the last half of 1929, the group contested the assessment on the grounds that the hospital was a nonprofit, charitable institution not subject to property taxes. The dispute was settled when ownership of the hospital was transferred to a new Minnesota nonprofit, also called Nicollet Hospitals, Inc., on March 27, 1934.

seven hundred hospitals had failed in the ten years following 1928. Nor did Eitel entirely escape the hard times, losing money between 1931 and 1933. But despite the hardships of the Depression years, the group's gamble in 1929 to purchase the hospital had generally worked to the benefit of the clinic. As chronicler of group practice C. Rufus Rorem reported in 1937, "The arrangements [with the hospital] had proved valuable . . . in conserving the time and energies of the staff in the treatment of hospitalized cases."[58]

But as the years went by, the relationship between the clinic and the hospital board grew less and less comfortable. Although Nicollet Hospitals, Inc., the nonprofit organization that owned Eitel Hospital, reserved ten of its fifteen board of trustee seats for members of the Nicollet Clinic, these seats were largely held by the increasingly conservative older members of the clinic who had made the original investment to purchase the hospital. Most of this group had cultivated an abiding faith in Alfred Stasel based on his success in guiding the hospital and clinic through the Depression and, as a result, took little interest in exercising day-to-day control of the hospital. But as the years passed and styles of management changed, Stasel lost the confidence of the new generation of leadership at the clinic.

Run like a proprietary hospital during a time of rapid hospital cost inflation, Eitel began to lag behind. Without an active and influential community board, its access to private donations was limited. By 1951, the Nicollet Clinic Board noted the "progressive deterioration in quality of service and morale," and, as a result, the hospital was "losing the support of our professional staff."[59]

But the difficulties the clinic was having with the hospital in the early 1950s were not serious enough to abandon the long-held vision of an "integrated hospital/clinic workshop."[60] After rejecting the King Cole Hotel as unsuitable in 1948, and the Blaisdell site as too expensive in 1952, the clinic, in the spring of 1953, began exploring the construction of a medical building adjacent to Eitel Hospital on the corner of Grant and Willow streets. The new medical building was part of a planned renovation of the hospital.

Financing the combined hospital renovation and medical building plan proved difficult. With a board dominated by physicians, the local hospital charity programs were reluctant to include Eitel in their recipient pool. This left private debt financing as the primary source of building funds. Debt financing, however, was made more difficult by the fact that a third party owned the land under the hospital. The clinic had never exercised its option to purchase the land, one of the many dreams smashed by the Depression. The current owner of the ground lease, George Eitel, nephew and heir of Jeanette Eitel and an independent physician on the Eitel staff, refused to take a second position to a mortgage company, fearing the security of the lease would be jeopardized. Unable to negotiate the purchase of the lease, the medical building was dropped from the plan.

A modest renovation of Eitel Hospital was completed in 1954, but that was not enough to keep it competitive with other hospitals in the area. Rising costs and the changing nature of medical care demanded expansion.

With debt financing ruled out, the one option that remained was to participate in the United Hospital Fund. Organized in 1955, the United Hospital Fund enlisted community support to raise millions of dollars for hospital improvements in Minneapolis, but private hospitals were excluded. This meant that in order for Eitel Hospital to participate, it would have to transfer control to a community or church board. To this end, the Nicollet Clinic gave up its right to appoint the majority of hospital trustees in June 1956. In the same month, the trustees asked for and accepted Stasel's resignation (another condition of participation in the fund).

The hospital established a new lay board of prominent Minneapolis leaders—including the Rev. Rueben Youngdahl

A serious fire kindled in the dry branches of a Christmas tree roared through the Eitel Hospital lobby on Christmas Eve 1956, killing eight patients and closing the hospital. After a dramatic, round-the-clock clean-up effort, the hospital reopened on February 3, 1957. Although no charges were ever brought against the hospital, the fire exposed several long-running battles between the hospital and various city departments, including the fire marshal. These revelations added to the public embarrassment the fire caused the hospital and, by its close association, the Nicollet Clinic as well.

of Mt. Olivet Lutheran Church—in March 1957. The Nicollet Clinic retained a single representative on the board. In June 1957, Nicollet Hospitals, Inc., was dissolved in favor of the new community hospital board. Construction of a new five-story wing, approved and financed in large part by the United Hospital Fund, began in September 1958.

For many of the physicians of the Nicollet Clinic, the resolution of the hospital situation came as a great relief. The vision of the integrated hospital/clinic had never been truly realized for a variety of reasons, both large and small. The expansion of the hospital projected in the 1929 ground lease had been delayed more than twenty years, first by the Depression and then by the inability of the hospital/clinic leadership to fully articulate or implement the vision. Years of energy that might have been spent building a new, modern home for the clinic and recruiting the best young physicians to fill the new offices had been spent drawing up plans for buildings that couldn't be financed, negotiating with a reluctant leaseholder, and accommodating an administration out of touch with the times. Relieved of indirect management responsibility, most of the Nicollet Clinic physicians continued to use Eitel for a majority of their cases, and the two organizations maintained a spirit of close collaboration for another twenty-five years.

BLAISDELL SITE REVISITED

With the option of building adjacent to the hospital finally closed and the ownership and expansion of Eitel Hospital resolved, the Nicollet Clinic partners decided in 1957 to make another offer to buy the Blaisdell Avenue lot. Their offer of $70,000 was immediately rejected by the owner, whose patience was rewarded in November when the two parties agreed on a purchase price of $100,000, the original asking price in 1952. With the decision where to build settled, the Nicollet Clinic was ready to abandon the shell that had comfortably restrained its growth for nearly forty years.

A CLINIC IN TRANSITION

The decade following World War II was a transitional era for the Nicollet Clinic. An initial period of rapid growth and energy following the return of the clinic's veterans was followed by a much longer period of consolidation. The Nicollet Avenue offices were old-fashioned and cramped, which made adding new physicians difficult. The many retirements during the 1950s made active recruitment essential; but, in spite of the reorganization in the late 1930s, the financial, practice, and management structures at the clinic made it increasingly difficult to attract talented young physicians to the group.

As is typical of many maturing organizations, a certain "us-and-them" feeling had developed between the old-guard partners and the new physicians just starting out. The founding physicians had been trained through apprenticeships with the distinguished physicians of their day, and many of the attitudes of this style of training had survived within the clinic into the 1950s. In the words of Arthur Ide, a surgeon who joined the clinic in 1951 and became a partner in 1955, new physicians served "in a very subordinate position . . . we were treated like residents. I stayed because I still had some idealism about group practice [and because] it was a challenge to make something out of the clinic."

The compensation system, to take another often-mentioned example, emphasized the physician's bookings-average over five years, a comfortable formula for the older partners. Distribution percentages were adjusted yearly to mixed reviews. But in the inflationary postwar period, the formula made it difficult to offer competitive salaries. Thus,

Many people contributed their special talents to the success of the Nicollet Clinic. One of these was Gertrude Stewart. Nicknamed "Skeeter" by S. Marx White for her petite size and enormous energy, she joined the clinic as registrar when it opened in 1921. Early on, in the absence of a full-time business manager, Stewart had assumed responsibility for hiring nurses and laboratory and X-ray staff, for purchasing, and, perhaps most importantly, for tracking bookings. With all this on her plate, it's no wonder she seemed to be "buzzing from one person or place to another," as Bob Newell remembered. She remained with the clinic as manager of the nonprofessional staff until retiring in the mid-1960s.

in spite of the often-expressed desire to increase the size of the clinic, the group added a net of only two physicians between 1947 and 1957. This returned the clinic to its pre-Depression staff size of nineteen full-time physicians.

By the mid-1950s, it was clear that the partnership structure was inhibiting the intentions of the group to create a permanent institution capable of growth. The administrative board was authorized to study the possibility of reorganizing as a professional association. Minnesota physician licensing laws, however, had been interpreted to prohibit physician groups from incorporating for the practice of medicine. By 1958 the decision to reorganize had been made, but no action could be taken until the Minnesota legislature changed the rules.

As the Nicollet Clinic administrative leaders struggled to meet the challenges of the organization, the individuals within the group went about the quieter business of providing excellent medical care and leadership within the medical community. With a new facility on the horizon, the Nicollet Clinic was poised and ready to move into the 1960s with renewed confidence and optimism.

4

A NEW ERA
THE NICOLLET CLINIC 1957 TO 1972

THE 1960S OFFERED TREMENDOUS OPPORTUNITY FOR expanding the Nicollet Clinic. The cold war with the Soviet Union and hotter military action in Vietnam kept government spending at near-World War II levels, priming an economy no longer restrained by the materials shortages of the early postwar period. Real interest rates were at all-time-low levels and the nation's economy was growing rapidly. Optimism about the future was the order of the day; it was a time to challenge the frontiers of space, expand the reach of American influence, and push forward in the battle against disease, disability, and injustice.

Each week seemed to produce new and astonishing surgical and medical treatments. The Sabin oral polio vaccine, widely distributed in 1962, eliminated the fear of polio; the measles vaccine was introduced in 1963. Society celebrated physicians and the achievements of medicine as never before. Huge television audiences tuned in every week to watch medical dramas such as *Ben Casey, Doctor Kildare*, and *The Nurses*.[61] This extraordinary interest in medicine helped to create a nation of medical care consumers who were "unorganized but as an aggregate prone to medicalize [their] problems and to press for increasing the availability of health services."[62] Medicare, introduced

S. Marx White became one of the oldest practicing physicians in the Twin Cities. He remained deeply committed to the success of the clinic he had founded, serving as a member of the emeritus staff after his retirement in 1952. He continued to see a small number of patients and consult with the staff until just a few months before his death in 1966 at age ninety-three.

in 1966, socialized the cost of hospitalization for elders and created "a bonanza" for the medical profession.[63]

BUILDING A NEW HOME

In the fall of 1957, Ellerbe and Associates began preliminary design work for the new Nicollet Clinic at the corner of Blaisdell and Franklin avenues. Various clinics were visited during the design process, including the Dakota Clinic in Fargo, also designed by Ellerbe, and the St. Louis Park Medical Center. After a year of planning, a final design was approved in January 1959. The Minneapolis general contractor Kraus-Anderson Company began construction the following November.

To own and manage the new building, the group set up a real estate holding company, the Nicollet Real Estate Corporation. Incorporated in February 1959, its membership was restricted to partners of the Nicollet Clinic, each holding roughly equal shares in the corporation. A twenty-year bond issue was offered to help raise necessary construction funds. In keeping with his long years of commitment to the group, S. Marx White was the first to respond to the bond offering.

Construction moved forward uneventfully at first, but it soon became clear that a few of the partners were less than firmly committed to the new building. Wallace Nelson, then the elected head of the partnership, became convinced that the entire project should be reevaluated and on at least one occasion called a halt to construction. Robert Newell, who as Business Manager was overseeing the administrative details of the construction project, looked to the other members of the Building Committee—Asher White and Arthur Ide—for assistance in addressing Nelson's concerns. With some effort, the committee kept the project on track and on schedule.

The finishing touches were put on the building during the summer of 1960. On September 26, 1960, after a weekend move, the Nicollet Clinic opened at 2001 Blaisdell Avenue. Laid out in the shape of a Maltese cross, the one-story building presented a facade of Indiana limestone and light brick to Blaisdell Avenue. A public wing housed the entrance lobby and reception area, the business office, and the pharmacy. The central reception desk directed patients into the other three wings housing the various departments and examining rooms. The building contained sixty examining rooms, and the parking lot had space for sixty-five cars. With an eye toward the rapidly expanding demand for medical care, the group had directed Ellerbe to reinforce the building's foundation to carry an additional three stories.

Nineteen physicians, three more than were present on opening day in 1921, made the move to the new offices. The nonphysician staff of forty-five, however, was two-and-one-half times as large as it had been in 1921, an indication of how much the practice of medicine had changed in the intervening years. In the words of Howard L. Horns, who had joined the internal medicine department in 1955, "It was a good building, and still is. . . . It really functioned quite well."

"ONE OF THE HARDEST TIMES"

The prospect of new space allowed the clinic to conclude negotiations with four new physicians, each of whom would provide the clinic with long service and leadership. Internist Thomas M. Recht joined the staff in July 1960, and Donald G. Velleck, another internist, followed six months later. Ann W. Arnold and Marie Moorhead, partners in a private obstetrics and gynecology practice in downtown Minneapolis, arrived in February 1961.

The joy of working in a new, spacious, and well-designed medical building was dimmed somewhat by the news that the group was suffering financially in early 1961. Collections in January were the lowest in three years. This, combined with increased expenses, presented a serious financial problem.[64] Robert Newell speculated that many patients, seeing the brand-new facility, may have adopted the attitude "My gosh they've got so darn much money I can put off paying the bill for a month or two." Collections did begin to rebound by April, although not soon enough for Arthur Ide. Elected president of the administrative board in February, Ide's first job was to notify the partners that they would miss a paycheck in March.

Had this been the only problem to fall in his lap, Ide would probably not remember 1961 as "one of the hardest times." Shortly before Ide's election, however, Newell resigned as the clinic's business manager. When internal struggles over the construction of the building turned into arguments over how the new space would be used, Newell decided he had had enough.[65]

The clinic board, with one of its newest members as chair, was faced with navigating the group through their first full year in the new building without a business manager. Wishing to save money and believing that they could manage the operation of the clinic through committees, board members voted to eliminate the position of business manager. This, according to Howard Horns, was a doomed decision, leading to a period "characterized by frequent, almost daily meetings—many of extended length—sometimes interrupted so that the partners could practice medicine for a few hours."[66]

A PROFESSIONAL ASSOCIATION

To the credit of Arthur Ide, the various crises in finance and personnel were not allowed to derail the long-planned reorganization of the partnership when the opportunity arose. Early in 1961, the Minnesota Medical Association approved a bill creating a new class of medical group, the professional association. This "blessing" cleared the way for legislative reform of the rules governing "corporate medicine."

Howard Horns, then serving as a member of the State Board of Medical Examiners and one of the authors of the bill, explained the need this way: "The question came up about the formation of [tax-deferred] retirement funds. Medicine kept running into trouble with the IRS. In order to satisfy the IRS it was necessary to form a corporation. . . . But there was a state law preventing the corporate practice of medicine, so we had to write a new law."

The Minnesota Professional Corporation Act was passed in May 1961. Among other things, it provided the mechanism by which groups of three or more physicians could incorporate as a professional association and thereby centralize management and perpetuate the group. Incorporation provided numerous tax benefits, allowing benefits previously paid out of a partner's taxable income, such as insurance premiums and death benefits, to be treated as deductible business expenses for the corporation and untaxed benefits to the employee. The new law also cleared the way for the development of tax-sheltered employee pension plans for the former partners who were ineligible to participate in such plans.[67]

As soon as the bill passed, the group moved forward to incorporate the Nicollet Clinic as a professional association. The final draft of the bylaws was approved in January 1962, to take effect in April of that year. The new structure provided for a five-member board of directors, each serving staggered three-year terms. The board, elected by the members of the association, chose its own officers. In recognition of the focus on stimulating growth, "Staffing and Recruiting" was the single standing committee. Department heads would function as a committee whenever clinical practice policy decisions were necessary.

All shareholders were required to be licensed to practice medicine in Minnesota and board-certified in their specialties. Each would own an equal share in the Nicollet Clinic Professional Association. Members reaching the age of seventy could continue their association with the clinic as nonvoting "emeritus staff" members. Continuing its tradition of rotating the presidency, the board named Fred A. Rice as the first president of the new organization.

Although the new business structure satisfied the state, the Internal Revenue Service (IRS), worried over the loss of revenues, continued to question the tax status of physician groups. In the spring of 1968, the IRS challenged the Nicollet Clinic's corporate status, demanding past taxes be paid by the group as a partnership. The IRS action was part of a nationwide effort to roll back the growing tide of medical groups operating as incorporated and unincorporated associations, including the St. Louis Park Medical Center, which was also facing an IRS challenge. After numerous losses in court, however, the IRS relented in the fall of 1969, before the Nicollet Clinic's case could be heard in court.

MANAGING FOR GROWTH

The months in 1961 when the partnership handled its affairs without a business manager left no doubt about the scope and importance of the job. At the suggestion of Howard Horns, William T. Middlebrook, recently retired as chief administrator of the University of Minnesota, was brought in as a business consultant to the group. Middlebrook, a mild-mannered man with a forceful personality and a talent for putting ideas together and presenting them logically, found the group more than ready to accept a more disciplined management style.

Middlebrook's first move was to recommend William Costello, a graduate of the university's business school who had twelve years of management experience, as the new business manager. Costello began work in July 1962, preparing the group for the new management systems he and Middlebrook were about to introduce, systems that could more effectively support the closely coordinated work of a growing multispecialty group practice.

Originally hired to help the group reorganize, William Middlebrook continued to work with the Nicollet Clinic for more than ten years. "He was a marvelous person," Howard Horns remembers. "He had a great sense of humor and would liven up the whole place. Introducing Middlebrook was the best day's work I did for the clinic."

In August, Middlebrook presented the group with a detailed report. The principal objective, he wrote, was "through delegation, to relieve the Board of Directors of the necessity of dealing with day-to-day operating problems on a piecemeal, ad hoc basis." This would require organization, a written code of policy, and a realistic budget informed by long-range planning in all departments.

Not limiting his analysis to the organization of the business office, Middlebrook noted that "the medical specialties are physically grouped, but . . . the physicians function organizationally on an individual basis, rather than departmentally, by specialties." He warned the group that the "present confusion will persist until there exists organization on the medical side which will sift and channel medical problems and needs to the business manager."[68] It was time, he told the group, to appoint a chief of medical services to handle the day-to-day medical administration problems now handled on a "piecemeal" basis.

There were, Middlebrook concluded, several major tasks that needed to be completed concurrently with the management reorganization. First, the building was underutilized, which indicated the need to redouble efforts to recruit physicians. The promised benefit package—retirement pensions and the like—needed implementation. Finally, in line with the founders' strong academic ties, Middlebrook recommended that the clinic's university-based teaching programs be strengthened and supported through the creation of a nonprofit foundation.[69]

Middlebrook's prescription for organizational renewal was embraced wholeheartedly by the group. Costello and his staff immediately began to prepare a detailed report on the current and future use of the building. Budgeting and long-range planning were implemented in all departments by the end of 1963. Howard Horns was appointed chief of medical services, a position he held until 1971. By April 1963, Middlebrook and Costello had a pension plan in place and had revised the compensation formula to more accurately reflect both the contribution of individual physicians and their department's share of the overhead. The Nicollet Clinic Foundation was created soon after in August 1963.

REAPING THE REWARDS

The management overhaul, outlined by Middlebrook and implemented by Costello and Horns, quickly began to pay dividends. The comprehensive budgets and detailed plans, for instance, cut the number of administrative meetings from a high of three per week in 1961 to twelve to fifteen per year by the end of 1963, thus conserving physician time for patient care.

In accord with Middlebrook's recommendations, the clinic implemented its first long-range planning process in 1962, setting as a main goal the doubling of the physician staff by 1970. To meet this goal, recruiting was pushed to the top of the agenda and entrusted to Howard Horns. During 1963 and 1964, Horns recruited one psychologist and five physicians, including internist A. Sigrid Gilbertsen. Donald Velleck, the next chair of the staffing committee, matched Horns' record in 1967, adding six physicians to the clinic in one year.

Over the decade, internal medicine, the largest department, grew by four physicians. Mental health programs expanded to include three psychologists and a speech therapist. An ophthalmologist was added in 1965 and a vascular/thoracic surgeon in 1970. Nevertheless, the clinic did not meet the goal of doubling its physician staff. By the end of the decade, the clinic included twenty-eight physicians—only nine more than had moved into the Blaisdell office in 1960. In a retrospective history of the clinic, Howard Horns wrote that the "acquisition of a new staff was not easy because of vigorous competition from other multispecialty clinics and single specialty clinics which for a period of time appeared more desirable to many specialists finishing training."[70] William Costello attributed the slower-than-expected growth to a general shortage of physicians during this period.

But to focus on the size of the physician staff as the main indicator of growth is to miss a critical fact. The business of the clinic more than doubled during the 1960s. From 1959 to 1970, patient revenues jumped from $711,000 to $1.8 million. New-patient registrations, another common measure of clinic growth, grew from 4,625 to 8,613 during the same period. The business fundamentals of the group were clearly well established.

NICOLLET CLINIC FOUNDATION

By 1970, the clinic supported two clinical education programs. The pediatrics department offered an in-office teaching program for university medical students. Under the guidance of pediatrician Northrop Beach, students learned how to examine children and talk to mothers, as well as the basics of clinical pediatrics. Also, the psychiatry department created an internship program in the clinical practice of psychology. Its first intern, Ralph Underwager, joined the group in 1967 after completing his doctorate, pointing the way to an effective strategy for recruiting physicians—"Teach and you shall find."

This sort of educational activity fell under the auspices of the newly created Nicollet Clinic Foundation. The foundation's mission, articulated by William Middlebrook, was to be "the engine for, or at least the facilitator for, continuing education, continuing research, and writing."[71] A clinic-sponsored series of "Fall Seminars," begun in 1965, was one of the first projects of the foundation. The seminars, held once a year for the next several years at the Leamington Hotel, showcased the work of the specialists of the Nicollet Clinic. A nationally known speaker was usually invited to give a keynote address, with a scientific program presented by members of the clinic staff.[72]

The Nicollet Clinic Foundation, managed by William Costello, raised money primarily from clinic staff and through a number of bequests from grateful patients. With no full-time staff or endowment, the foundation stayed small and concentrated on providing small grants to physicians and others within the clinic who were doing research projects. A survey of the characteristics of incoming neurotic patients, a research project of John Powers, Ph.D., typifies the kind of work supported during the second half of the 1960s. "[The foundation] wasn't high on the priority list," Costello noted. "It was the kind of thing that [would have] needed more champions." Lacking a solid champion within the organization, the foundation became inactive in 1970 when new tax-code rules increased the paperwork load on nonprofits.

NICOLLET CLINIC PHARMACY

The pharmacy that had been loosely affiliated with the Nicollet Clinic since 1921, and owned by a group of its physicians and Alfred Stasel since 1933, had moved with the group to the new building on Blaisdell Avenue. Ownership in the pharmacy was by 1962 limited to a relatively small subset of older physicians, the pharmacist Roy A. Carlson, and a few people outside the clinic. As the next generation took leadership of the clinic, old arguments over the ethics of physicians owning the pharmacy resurfaced.

A reorganization plan put together by Middlebrook and

Costello called for bringing the pharmacy under the direct control of the group. After a few more years of debate and negotiation, the Nicollet Clinic Professional Association purchased the pharmacy in 1966. Consolidating ownership enabled the group to operate the pharmacy in a manner that avoided any individual benefit or the appearance of an incentive to prescribe within the clinic. Having a pharmacy on the premises was seen as a convenience for the clinic's patients if they chose to use it, but, as Costello observed, "If the pharmacy was in the clinic building, the clinic would be held responsible for it, and that being the case, we felt strongly that the clinic should own and control it."

The restructured pharmacy was able to reduce prices charged to patients for maintenance drugs by 15 to 20 percent. Tighter management also reduced the prices of drugs and supplies sold directly to the Nicollet Clinic, while at the same time improving the net profit of the pharmacy. In 1969, the pharmacy was renamed the Nicollet Clinic Pharmacy, replacing the long-used name Allied Apothecary.

GROWING UP AND OUT

Under the leadership of Howard Horns, William Middlebrook, and William Costello, the group continued to improve the administrative and business systems of the clinic. Business was increasing rapidly at the Blaisdell office, expanding much faster than the physician staff. As staff shortages became more difficult, the group decided to close the Richfield pediatrics office. Northrop Beach argued against this decision, feeling it would be a major inconvenience to his patients, and extracted a pledge that a new suburban medical office would be opened in the near future to fill the gap. The group began looking for office space in Bloomington in 1966, but the project was displaced in 1967 by the decision to expand the office on Blaisdell Avenue first.

The younger staff at the Nicollet Clinic influenced the decision to open a satellite office in the early 1970s. According to Max Boller, an internist who joined the clinic in 1968, "I think the young people were anxious for some autonomy in our practice. . . . Essentially, all of the younger people moved to the Burnsville office, part-time, and we established a call schedule there."

The addition of a second story in 1968 doubled the size of the Blaisdell Avenue building. H. Westin and Associates, which provided the combined architectural and construction services for the new space, retained the cut-limestone and light-brick-exterior facade and added a terrazzo mural to the Blaisdell Avenue entry. Although part of the new space was initially left unfinished, the growing practice soon occupied the entire second floor.

With the expansion of the main building out of the way, the possibility of establishing a network of suburban primary care clinics came under discussion. The population of the suburban rings was beginning to explode, and the clinic realized it needed to follow its patients. Robert E. Olson, an internist who had joined the clinic in 1967, became the chair of the Area Offices Committee and began actively pursuing the objective. In April 1971, the board of directors decided to open "an office in the Burnsville area within the next several months."[73] A thorough search of the area located suitable office space at 151 West Burnsville Crosstown, and the new clinic—offering internal medicine, psychology, and pediatric services—opened to patients in August 1971.

In his annual report for 1971-72, Thomas Recht, who had succeeded Howard Horns as director of medical services, predicted that the new office would soon "be as profitable as the main clinic."[74] Indeed, combined new-patient registrations in 1972, the first full year of operation in Burnsville, were up by more than 3,000, after remaining between 7,000 and 8,000 for over eight years. The rented office in Burnsville, with only 1,200 square feet of space, had created a larger increase in new-patient registrations than the opening of the Blaisdell clinic had in 1960. The Nicollet Clinic was clearly heading in a new direction.

5

HMOS ARRIVE

THE NICOLLET CLINIC 1973 TO 1983

By 1970, MEDICINE HAD ENTERED ANOTHER PERIOD OF crisis. *Fortune* magazine, for instance, led its January issue with an editorial "It's Time to Operate," calling for "radical changes" to correct the "financial distortions, the inequities, and the managerial redundancies in the system."[75] As was the case in the 1930s and again in the 1950s, the rapidly growing cost and inequitable distribution of medical care was attracting mainstream attention. Large, prepaid group practices like the Kaiser Foundation Health Plan, the health and hospital services giant in California, were managing to control costs, and their success was being touted in the press and within the Nixon administration.

As the cost of medical care spiraled upward, the need for a predictable medical expense, without the threat of bankrupting medical bills as a result of sickness or accident, made prepayment more and more essential for consumers. To manage the huge potential risk and large cash flows, prepaid group plans contracted with insurance companies, who by the mid-1970s began creating their own health insurance plans. Over time, many different types of prepayment evolved—including private insurance health plans, nonprofit plans, consumer-owned plans, and private group practice plans, to name just a few.

For the Nicollet Clinic, it was simply time to try again to

Prepaid medical care refers to a contract between a health care provider and a patient (or between intermediaries for each). The provider, in exchange for a fee, promises to make a set package of medical care services available in the event the patient needs care. The earliest prepaid plans were industry-specific, created to provide medical care to workers. Most often, a specific group of physicians, either on contract or salary, provided the care, thus shifting some of the risk for a patient's health to the physician group. Because physicians had an incentive for keeping patients healthy and out of the hospital, early and preventive care were more likely under this system, which, in theory, held down medical costs.

implement a successful prepaid medical care plan. As early as 1933, the clinic had entered into serious discussions with the Post Office Employees Union in St. Paul to provide a range of medical and hospital services. The plan was hammered out over the course of a year and prepared for presentation to the Hennepin County Medical Society but was dropped in late 1934 before it got a hearing.

The clinic tried again in 1941, entering a provider agreement with Group Health Mutual as described in chapter 3. After the provider agreement with Group Health was discontinued, further experiments in prepaid care were largely abandoned until the late 1960s when the new leadership decided the time for prepaid medicine had arrived. The health maintenance organization (HMO), according to William Costello, "appeared to be an effective and powerful force in attracting and maintaining our patient population. Other HMOs were growing, the government was advocating the strategy, and, if you didn't belong to an HMO, you stood to see a good part of your patients disappear."

The close connection the group had maintained to Eitel Hospital led naturally to discussion of the possibilities of combining hospitalization and medical care under one shared-risk agreement. In the late 1960s, Jack Rivall, administrator of Eitel Hospital, could see that patients were deserting Eitel for better-equipped, larger hospitals such as Abbott Northwestern. Suburban patients were reluctant to come downtown unless they needed the specialized services of the larger teaching hospitals. The fortunes of Eitel Hospital depended heavily on the clinic—nearly 50 percent of its medical staff were Nicollet physicians. Consequently, Rivall and the Eitel Hospital Board were very interested in pursuing the creation of a health plan. By participating in a health maintenance organization with the Nicollet Clinic, Eitel would accept an equal share of the risk but, in return, gain an increased and more stable flow of patients.

In late 1968, Rivall and Howard Horns visited the Metropolitan Medical Center in Detroit, which had created an early HMO, to learn about the feasibility of combining hospital and medical coverage. On their return, Rivall talked with the Eitel Hospital people, and Horns talked with the clinic. Dr. Sigrid Gilbertsen became particularly interested in the HMO idea and with her energy and influence the idea gained support.[77]

The term "health maintenance organization" was coined in the early 1970s to describe a particular type of prepaid medical care and later came to be used for any organization offering comprehensive health care services to a defined group of people at a fixed periodic payment.[76] The term was brought into public usage by the Nixon administration, which adopted the health maintenance organization as its central weapon in the battle against rising health care costs.

A NEW HEALTH CARE PLAN

In March 1971, Gilbertsen, as chair of the Medical Practice Study Committee, presented the group with a plan to develop a nonprofit health services corporation with Eitel Hospital. By May her committee received approval from the clinic to borrow up to $25,000 to capitalize the corporation. Gilbertsen was elected chair of the founding board of the Nicollet-Eitel Family Health Plan.

Early in the development process, Blue Cross Blue Shield of Minnesota was approached to provide administrative and marketing services for the new HMO. After several months of negotiations and cooperative work in 1971, Blue Cross Blue Shield pulled out and was replaced by a commercial insurer, AETNA Life and Casualty Company AETNA, one of the insurance companies involved in creating the Harvard Community Health Plan in Boston a few years earlier, was interested in promoting the multiple-carrier-model prepaid health plan nationwide,[78] what is known in the 1990s as an exclusive provider plan.[79] With an administrative partner secured, the fledgling health plan hired its first executive director, Nicholas Spring, in 1972.[80]

The leadership of Gilbertsen and Recht, and the support of Horns, carried the group past their initial and quite natural reluctance to jump into the still very new field of HMOs. Although there was mild opposition, it was not

NICOLLET-EITEL FAMILY HEALTH PLAN FOUNDING BOARD, 1971

Sigrid Gilbertsen, M.D., Chair
William Costello
Frank Krause
Allan Moore
Thomas Recht, M.D.
Louis Regan
Fred Rice, M.D.
Jack Rivall
Paul Stewart, M.D.

enough to dampen the group's general enthusiasm for the project, which was to be only a small test plan with any losses shared by Eitel Hospital. Risk would be kept to a minimum by restricting the plan to employee groups.

By early 1972, the Nicollet-Eitel Family Health Plan was ready for approval by the state insurance commission. Unfortunately, the state had no experience with this sort of prepaid medical insurance plan and Insurance Commissioner Berton W. Heaton felt he did not have the statutory authority to regulate a policy that was not strictly indemnity insurance.[81] The start-up of the Nicollet-Eitel Family Health Plan was delayed for more than a year while the state got its regulatory apparatus in order.[82] A slightly modified plan was approved in July 1973, allowing AETNA to begin marketing to its Twin Cities client employers and national accounts. By the end of 1973, the new plan had about 650 members and was gaining momentum.

At about the same time the Nicollet Clinic was developing the Nicollet-Eitel Family Health Plan, St. Louis Park Medical Center was developing the Medcenter Health Plan. The two health plans were both early leaders in the local and national HMO movement. In contrast to the Medcenter Health Plan, the Nicollet-Eitel Family Health Plan was closely controlled by the Nicollet Clinic, which provided all of the primary medical service and most of the referral care needed by health plan members. The historically close relationship between Eitel Hospital and the Nicollet Clinic had made it possible to develop an HMO, which Dr. Paul Ellwood, an advisor to the Nixon administration, described in 1974 as "unique in the Midwest because the hospital shares with the Clinic the financial risk of the enterprise."[83] In addition, the Nicollet-Eitel Family Health Plan operated as a virtual division of the clinic.[84] This had certain advantages for the smaller group practice, chief among them that the growth of the plan could be more precisely managed, allowing the clinic to keep its facilities aligned with patient demand.

REVITALIZING THE PLAN

As early as 1973, the adm0inistrators of the Nicollet-Eitel Family Health Plan and the Medcenter Health Plan in St. Louis Park were informally discussing plans for joint marketing and an eventual merger, driven in part by the desire to accommodate the larger employers who were looking for an HMO option with a broad geographic reach. The possibility of merging resurfaced in 1976 when growth of the Nicollet-Eitel Family Health Plan had slowed to the point where it had become a financial drain on both Eitel Hospital and the Nicollet Clinic. The Nicollet Clinic's Thomas Recht, William Costello, and A. Charles Bredesen, a consultant to the plan, took a proposal to merge the two health plans to the leadership of St. Louis Park Medical Center. After considerable discussion, the message came back from the medical center that it was interested in the merger only if the two clinics also merged. The "deal killer," from the Nicollet Clinic's perspective, was the insistence of the St. Louis Park Medical Center Board that it be given the right to accept or reject beneficiary status for each of the Nicollet Clinic physicians. In effect this meant that, rather than accepting whoever might be on the Nicollet Clinic staff, St. Louis Park Medical Center wanted the right to assess each physician's work and accept or reject the physician for membership accordingly.

With no interest in accepting these terms, the Nicollet Clinic Board decided to rejuvenate the health plan on its own and asked Bredesen to go back to the drawing board to prepare a new marketing plan. Several weeks later, and still a consultant, Bredesen presented his recommendations. He was immediately offered the job of executive director of the Nicollet-Eitel Health Plan, which Nick Spring had resigned from about six months earlier.[85] Bredesen's only condition for accepting the offer was that he be given more leeway to operate independently of the clinic.[86]

Health maintenance organizations were attractive to consumers because they were relatively inexpensive and presented a generous set of benefits. They were inexpensive because they were selectively marketed to healthy people who worked for major corporations and, for at least the first ten years, the dollars coming in from membership growth were more than enough to offset the actual cost of providing services. HMOs were not intended to control costs over the long-term and, indeed, were not capable of doing so. For the Nicollet-Eitel Family Health Plan and for the Medcenter Health Plan, the HMO was a strategy for growth, for keeping patients, and for providing a steady income for the groups. On the national level, it was a strategy to head off a nonprofit national health plan that would cover everybody with a uniform set of benefits.

"I remember watching Dr. [Sigrid] Gilbertsen. She was an excellent physician and a very bright woman, but she had a real gruff appearance. She had been sitting there the whole time with her head down listening to my upbeat talk [about marketing the health plan]. Finally, while we were going over some questions, she looks up and says, 'Well, if it's so damn easy why don't you do it?' That was my job offer."

Charles Bredesen

An analysis of the plan's membership showed that over two-thirds were single adults living in Minneapolis. The plan did not, by underwriting standards, have enough families in it. Thus, the first major change was the decision to implement a marketing strategy that favored the Burnsville office and targeted families. In addition, a decision was made to aggressively discount premiums for specific groups in order to attract a lower-utilizing, healthier group of employees. This break from community rating, where all groups are offered the same premium/benefits package, was a first, according to Bredesen, and was soon followed by the rest of the market.

The increased energy and marketing self-confidence paid off. By 1981, enrollments had grown to almost 19,000 from 3,000 in 1976. Bookings from the health plan had grown to 35 percent of the clinic's total gross bookings, from $229,000 in 1976 to $3.3 million in the early 1980s.[87]

ADDING CLINICS

The tiny satellite office on the Burnsville Crosstown, which had opened in 1971, grew quickly, from 1,200 to 3,200 square feet in less than a year. In 1974, encouraged by the community's acceptance of the new clinic, the Nicollet Clinic Board of Directors approved a plan to close the Crosstown office and build a larger office on the Fairview Ridges Hospital Campus, also in Burnsville. This plan was set aside when leased space on the Fairview Ridges Campus became available. Another location was added when Dr. Charles Zinn of Wayzata asked the group to assume his practice in November 1976. The Nicollet Clinic was now operating in three offices—Minneapolis, Burnsville, and Wayzata—housing a total of thirty-three physicians.

After the HMO was reenergized in 1977, the pressure to add satellite offices in growing, demographically attractive areas increased. Charles Bredesen took the lead, urging the clinic to plan offices in Bloomington, Eagan, Rosemount, and downtown Minneapolis. Bredesen told the board that 1978 would be a "critical year" for HMOs, as many of the larger businesses in the western suburban ring were making plans to offer HMO benefit options to their employees for the first time.

In early 1978, the shareholders approved moving ahead with a new office in Bloomington. Located at 80th and Xerxes, the office opened in September 1979 in leased space. It was an immediate success.

Financing this expansion, however, proved difficult. The war on inflation, led by Paul Volker and the Federal Reserve, had driven interest rates to nearly 20 percent. But the solid success of the satellite offices in attracting patients to the clinic kept the board of directors and William Costello searching for creative ways to finance continued growth. It was not an easy task. Convincing a group of physicians in the 1970s to use retained earnings, or internal capital, to finance growth was akin to asking them to chain themselves to the clinic for the next five or so years. Money spent opening a satellite office in Burnsville or Bloomington came out of funds that otherwise would have been available to compensate the physicians. As Bredesen explained, "If that leads to a big increase in patient volume for the clinic in ten years, that doesn't do the individual physician any good if (a) your practice is full already, or (b) you are not still at the clinic to collect."

Thomas Recht, an advocate of expanding both the technical ability and geographic reach of the clinic, often confronted the group's unwillingness to use retained earnings to finance expansion: "They would not set aside X amount of money for capital improvements, so everything was debt financed. . . . Everyone wanted the last penny paid out of the bottom line."

By 1980, the leased office space at Fairview Ridges was overloaded. It was time to build a larger Burnsville clinic.

As part of a strategy to finance the construction of a new building, Costello proposed a complex plan that would also fix another problem associated with success. As the value of clinic assets had increased over time, it had become increasingly difficult to maintain equal ownership of the real estate among the permanent staff. Costello's solution refinanced the Blaisdell office and created a partnership, Nicollet Clinic Properties, to purchase and hold the assets. The change would allow the older members to realize some of their gains and move back to a lower base, thereby making it much easier for new physicians to buy in.[88] To make it happen, the board approved $1.9 million in new borrowing on the Blaisdell office and the creation of the property partnership in the late summer of 1980.

After a very difficult year of delays due in part to the poor financial market, the partnership was able to arrange $3.4 million in tax-free financing for the new Burnsville satellite at Fairview Ridges through the sale of municipal bonds underwritten by AETNA.[89] Construction of the 40,000-square-foot clinic, designed by Ellerbe and Associates, began in the spring of 1982.

The difficulties arranging financing for construction did not halt the geographic expansion of the Nicollet Clinic into leased office space. A satellite office in Eagan opened in late 1981. In March 1981, plans were made for moving the Wayzata office to Ridgedale Shopping Mall in Minnetonka. The 6,800-square-foot office opened on Ridgedale Drive in May 1982, one month before the St. Louis Park Medical Center moved its Ridgedale office to a new location just down the street.

The Nicollet Clinic's Bloomington office introduced a new concept in ambulatory care in mid-1982. The "Urgicare Center" was developed to meet the logical imperatives of the health maintenance organization and offered extended office hours and walk-in convenience to the community. "You have to provide the services you advertise," said Tom Recht, "which meant easy access and access at odd hours."

Initially, the Minnesota Emergency Physicians Association (MEPA) staffed the Urgicare Center, until the Nicollet Clinic took over staffing in July 1983. The Urgicare Center was part of a national movement toward free-standing ambulatory care clinics, of which only fifty-five existed in 1978. By 1982, six hundred had been created nationally, with patient volume growing by 20 percent each year.[90]

Nicollet-Eitel Health Plan managers were among the first to begin developing and managing HMOs for other physician groups, arranging contracts to provide these services in the late 1970s to the Midelfort Clinic in Eau Claire, the Jackson Clinic in Madison, and the Nicolet Clinic in Neenah, all in Wisconsin. These contracts had little support back at the clinic, however. "We had no objection per se," said Tom Recht, recalling the attitude of the group. "But why? We're struggling to build our resources here. Don't waste your resources all over the country."

PRELUDE TO A MERGER

In spite of the remarkable turnaround of the Nicollet-Eitel Health Plan and the rapid expansion of the Nicollet Clinic after 1976, a growing list of market forces was working against smaller health care providers. The health care market was driving HMOs toward a broader array of services and benefit plans. Medicare plans, dental plans, and patient education and health promotion all required expensive start-up investments and a large patient base to sustain them. The Nicollet-Eitel plan had implemented all of these programs but was growing increasingly worried that the growth rate needed to sustain this level of activity was out of reach. "For a plan of our size we were more actively involved in expanding the scope of our services than anyone," Bredesen recalled. "But we were stretched very thinly and the only way we could make the long-term plan work was to grow at a disproportionate rate, and that was going to require more offices, hours, patient services, and marketing expenditures than we were able to afford."

The Nicollet Clinic's relationship with Eitel Hospital had also become a limiting factor. For more than fifty years the Nicollet Clinic staff had provided the bulk of the patients to Eitel Hospital. The Nicollet-Eitel Health Plan was one of the positive results of this long-term collaboration. But Eitel Hospital was in 1929, and remained in 1979, a community hospital, with a limited presence in the marketplace. Certificate-of-need legislation, passed in 1972, severely limited Eitel's ability to grow as long as a surplus of hospital beds existed in the region, even if patient preference could be generated. In 1975, for example, facing the increased utilization created by the health plan, Eitel applied for authorization to add sixty beds. This request was slashed to fifteen beds before it was eventually approved.

As the technology of care exploded through the 1970s, Eitel fell behind its larger, better-endowed rivals. By 1976, cracks were beginning to show in the Nicollet Clinic's long-term loyalty to Eitel. The younger obstetricians and pediatricians wanted access to the modern equipment they had been trained to use, which was not available at Eitel. Dissatisfaction reached a peak in 1980 when the obstetrics and gynecology department at the Nicollet Clinic withdrew from Eitel Hospital, switching its patients to Abbott Northwestern. Eitel continued to lose ground as the primary provider of hospital care to the Nicollet-Eitel plan as physicians at the satellite offices began to seek ties with the newer and more convenient Fairview Ridges and Southdale hospitals. Contracts with these two hospitals became a significant part of Nicollet-Eitel hospitalization expenses by the early 1980s, which caused considerable irritation at Eitel. Unable to expand and losing a significant part of its patient base to the newer, suburban hospitals, Eitel Hospital was in no position to invest heavily in the expansion of the health plan it shared with the Nicollet Clinic.

Across town the only other group-practice-based HMO in the Twin Cities was responding to the same market forces. Medcenter Health Plan and St. Louis Park Medical Center, though they had made different decisions and were experiencing more rapid growth, were also being confronted daily with evidence that survival in the coming years would require a larger patient base. Nicollet Clinic Manager William Costello watched the two similar organizations going head-to-head in the marketplace and wondered, "Why should we be fighting each other? Why shouldn't we get together and do it up better?" As the pressure on both groups increased, it was only a matter of time before the issue of joining forces would be put on the table again.

Chapter 1

1 "125 Years of Service: A History of the Hennepin County Medical Society," *Bulletin of the Hennepin County Medical Society* 51(June 1980 anniversary supplement): 12.

2 S. Marx White, *Minnesota Doctor* (Unpublished manuscript, Minnesota Historical Society, 1966), 36.

3 Ibid., 23.

4 Ibid., 36.

5 Ibid.

6 Ibid.

7 Minutes of the Nicollet Clinic, May 25, 1920.

8 George Halsey Hunt and Marcus Goldstein, *Medical Group Practice in the U.S.*, pub. no. 77 (Washington, D.C.: Federal Security Agency, Public Health Service, 1951), 2.

9 White, *Minnesota Doctor*, 36.

10 White, *Minnesota Doctor*, 37-38.

11 A. Flexner, *Medical Education in the United States and Canada*, bulletin no. 4 (New York: Carnegie Foundation, 1910).

12 Articles of Incorporation of the Nicollet Clinic, October 14, 1920.

13 Ibid.

14 James A. Johnson and S. Marx White, "The Nicollet Clinic," *Group Practice* 9 (March 1960): (reprint).

15 Angus Morrison, Organizing Committee Notes of the Nicollet Clinic, October 8, 1920.

16 Johnson and White, "The Nicollet Clinic."

17 S. Marx White, "The Origin of the Nicollet Clinic" (Internal document read at the twenty-fifth anniversary dinner of the Nicollet Clinic, January 21, 1946), 6.

Chapter 2

18 John Bell Williams, "Report of Visit of Inspection to Mayo and Other Clinics" (Internal document of the McGuire Clinic, Richmond, Virginia, 1925), 9.

19 A. G. Stasel, "Keeping the Cost of Adequate Professional Service Within the Reasonable Ability of the Average Person to Pay," Proceedings, Ninth Annual Conference of Clinic Managers, Madison, Wisconsin, October 17-18, 1934, 1: 327. This organization was the forerunner of the Medical Group Management Association.

20 John P. Schneider, Annual Director's Address, The Nicollet Clinic, January 13, 1925.

21 Ibid.

22 Editors, "Group Practice—A Menace or a Blessing?" *JAMA* 76(February 12, 1921): 452.

23 Fishbein, 1947, cited in *Medical Groups in the United States—A Survey of Practice Characteristics*, edited by Penny Havelick (Chicago: American Medical Association, 1990).

24 Robert Newell, interview with author, June 14, 1993.

25 Mark Peacock (Unpublished history of Park Nicollet, Park Nicollet Medical Foundation, 1991).

26 James A. Johnson, Minutes of the Nicollet Clinic, October 20-21, 1921.

27 Johnson and White, "The Nicollet Clinic."

28 C. Rufus Rorem and John H. Musser, *Private Group Medical Service: The Economic and Professional Aspects of a Private Clinic in a Mid-western City* (Chicago: Julius Rosenwald Fund, 1937), 4.

29 Barbara Martin, *History of the Hennepin County Medical Society, 1855-1955* (Minneapolis: Hennepin County Medical Society, 1982),429.

30 A. G. Stasel, "Historical Brief—Eitel Hospital (Doctor's Memorial Hospital) 1929-1954" (Internal document of the Nicollet Clinic, 1955), 1.

31 Eitel Hospital Ground Lease—Indenture, Jeanette E. Eitel, Lessor and The Nicollet Clinic of Minneapolis, Inc., Tenant, March 5, 1929.

32 Johnson and White, "The Nicollet Clinic."

33 Paul Starr, *The Social Transformation of American Medicine* (New York: Basic Books, 1982), 270.

34 G. M. MacKenzie, et al., "Group Medicine: A Discussion of the Economics of Medical Care," *The Modern Hospital* 65(November 1945), 45.

35 Annual Financial Reports of the Nicollet Clinic, 1933.

36 Robert Newell, "Recollection of Clinic Stories of the Depression Days" (Unpublished manuscript, Park Nicollet, Park Nicollet Medical Foundation, 1992).

37 S. Marx White, "The Doctors Leisure," *Bulletin of the Hennepin County Medical Society* 4(January 10, 1933): 309.

38 Leonard Wilson, *Medical Revolution in Minnesota: A History of the University of Minnesota Medical School* (St. Paul: Midewinin Press, 1989), 291.

39 Martin, *History of the Hennepin County Medical Society*, 620.

40 Wilson, *Medical Revolution in Minnesota*, 273.

41 Kansas Obstetrical and Gynecological Society, April 8, 1939.

42 Ray F. Cochrane, "Our Senior Educators: Jennings Crawford Litzenberg, M.D.," *Minnesota Medicine* 46(July 1966): 1111.

43 Catherine Corson West, "Olga Sophie Hansen, M.D.," *Journal Lancet* 80(August 1960): 401.

44 Minutes of the Nicollet Clinic, February 25, 1924.

45 "Martyr to His Profession," *Minneapolis Daily Star*, December 28, 1926.
46 Walter Haven, interview with Mark Peacock, 1991.

Chapter 3
47 Minutes of the Nicollet Clinic, May 15, 1937.
48 S. Marx White, "Presidential Address American College of Physicians," *Annals of Internal Medicine* 5(1932): 1540.
49 Jennings C. Litzenberg, "Presidential Address, 66th Annual Meeting of the American Gynecological Society, Colorado Springs, Colorado, May 26-28, 1941" (Republished in *Nicollet Clinic Bulletin*, July 1941, 23).
50 Minutes of the Nicollet Clinic, November 16, 1948.
51 Group Health Mutual, the insurance cooperative that had created the Group Health Association, evolved into Group Health, Inc., a staff model health plan and group medical practice.
52 Private correspondence from Asher White to "Bain" (probably J. B. Carey), January 16, 1946.
53 Robert Newell, interview with author, June 14, 1993.
54 Minutes of the Nicollet Clinic, August 25, 1953.
55 Northrop Beach, interview with author, August 2, 1993.
56 Robert Newell, interview with author, June 14, 1993.
57 *125 Years of Service*, 21.
58 Rorem and Musser, *Private Group Medical Service*, 4.
59 Minutes of the Nicollet Clinic, August 9, 1951.
60 Minutes of the Nicollet Clinic, September 27, 1955. This idea was also present in the initial discussion of building a hospital, Minutes of the Nicollet Clinic, February 20, 1920.

Chapter 4
61 Rosemary Stevens, *In Sickness and In Wealth: American Hospitals in the Twentieth Century* (New York: Basic Books, 1989), 228.
62 Eliot Freidson, *Medical Work in America—Essays on Health Care* (New Haven, Conn.: Yale University Press, 1989), 243.
63 Starr, *Social Transformation of American Medicine*, 370.
64 Robert Newell, Minutes of the Nicollet Clinic, February 9, 1961.
65 Robert Newell, interview with author, June 14, 1993.
66 Howard Horns, "History of the Nicollet Clinic, 1960-1976" (Internal paper, undated), 1.
67 Jule M. Hannaford, "The Minnesota Professional Corporation Act," *Minnesota Medicine* 44(November 1961): 483.
68 William Middlebrook, "Clinic Organization and Operation" (Internal document, August 1962).
69 Ibid.

70 Howard Horns, "History of the Nicollet Clinic, 1960-1976" (Internal document, undated), 2.
71 William Middlebrook, "General Recomendations" (Internal document, 1964).
72 Donald Velleck, interview with author, January 12, 1995.
73 Minutes of the Nicollet Clinic, April 22, 1971.
74 Thomas Recht, Annual Report of the Nicollet Clinic, 1971-72.

Chapter 5
75 Editorial, "It's Time to Operate," *Fortune*, January 1, 1970, 79.
76 Katherine Hiduchenko, "HMO's and Cost Containment," *Minnesota Medicine* 66(November 1983): 701.
77 Howard Horns, interview with author, July 20, 1993.
78 The Harvard Community Health Plan was one of the early HMOs, as defined by the Nixon administration. It was sold like an insurance policy by a variety of agents, hence "multiple carrier." In other words, a variety of insurance companies would at any given time be authorized to represent and sell the policy to the businesses who were buying insurance for their employees—far and away the majority of health plans sold in the 1970s.
79 Charles Bredesen, interview with author, August 18, 1994.
80 Thomas Recht, Annual Report of the Nicollet Clinic, 1971-72.
81 Indemnity insurance refers to a type of insurance in which the subscriber documents a covered loss and the insurer reimburses the subscriber.
82 Charles Bredesen, interview with author, August 18, 1994.
83 Editorial, *Minneapolis Star*, June 7, 1975.
84 Charles Bredesen, interview with author, September 22, 1994.
85 "Family" was dropped from the title of the plan after 1976.
86 Charles Bredesen, interview with author, August 18, 1994.
87 Minutes of the Nicollet Clinic, August 4, 1980, and Annual Report of the Nicollet Clinic, 1981.
88 William Costello, interview with author, June 30, 1993.
89 William Costello, Annual Report of the Nicollet Clinic, 1981, and Costello, correspondence with James Toscano, October 28, 1992, 10.
90 Richard Reeves, "The Corporate Transformation of Minnesota Medicine," *Minnesota Medicine* 67(January 1984): 9.

Photo History
Part I

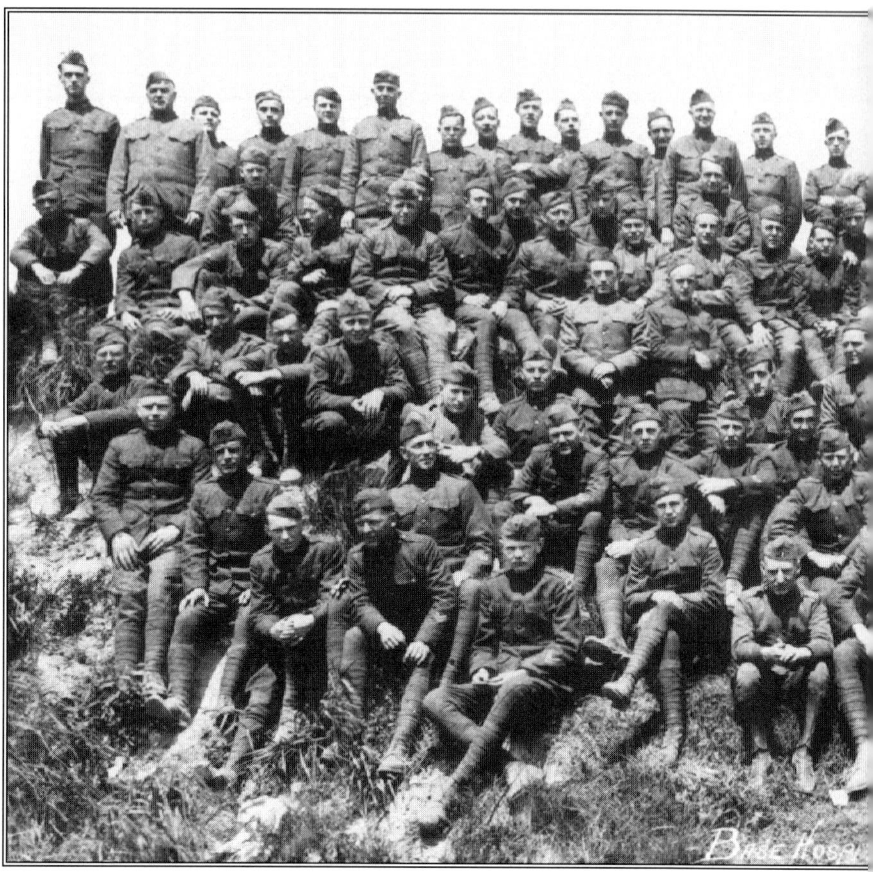

These members of the Base Hospital 26 unit served in France during World War I. The hospit was organized by the University of Minnesota Medical School in 1917 at the request of the U.S war department. Members were recruited from the staffs of the University of Minnesota and Mayo Clinic, and the community. The hospital's commissioned medical officers, including S. M White, organized it by specialty to best utilize the talents of physician staff.

Upon returning from the war, Drs. Gilbert Thomas and Angus Morrison resolved to pursu their idea of creating a group medical practice staffed by members of Base Hospital 26. Within years, the Nicollet Clinic group practice opened in downtown Minneapolis.

Photos from History of Base Hospital *26, © 1920 D.D. Gretchell, Minneapolis. Courtesy the University of Minnesota archives.*

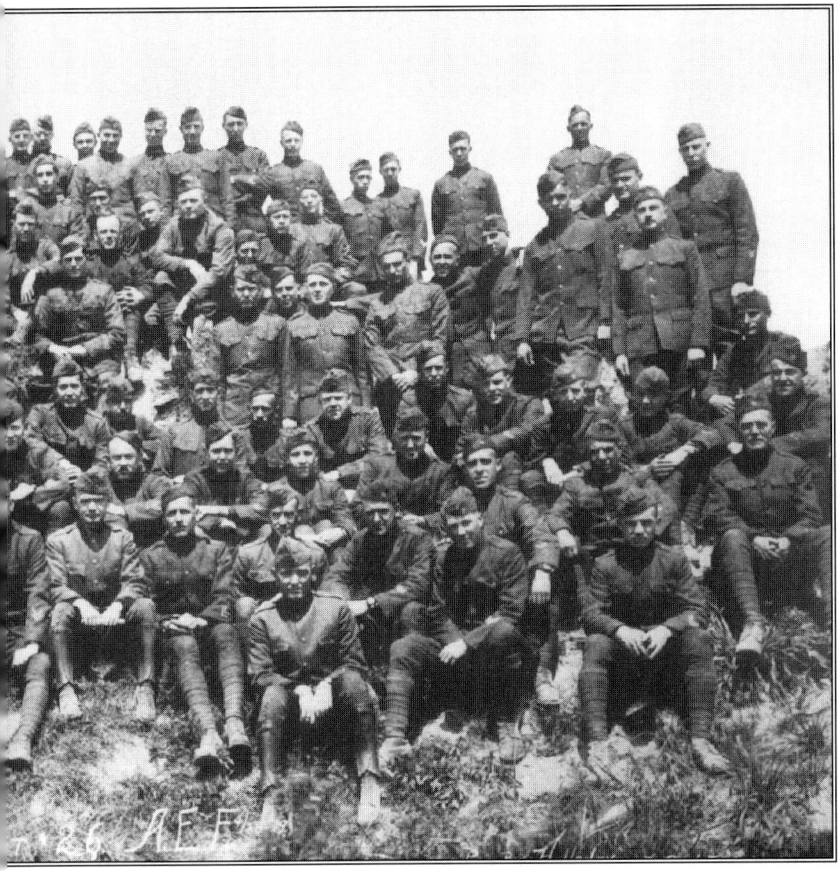

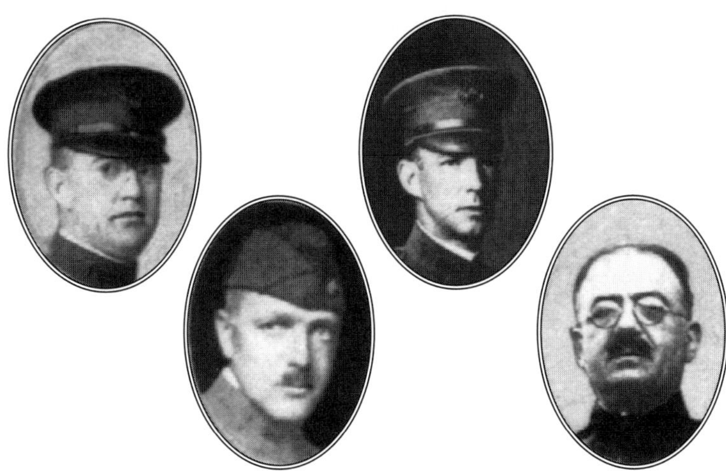

TOP
Major G. Thomas, Minneapolis
Captain A. Morrison, Minneapolis

BOTTOM
Major Charles Reed, Minneapolis
Major S. M. White, Minneapolis

Founders of the Nicollet Clinic January 25, 1921

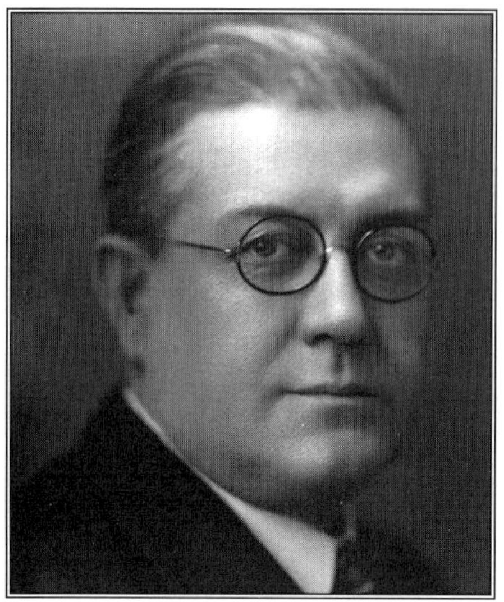

Jennings Crawford Litzenberg, M.D., 1870-1948; Obstetrics and Gynecology
Photo circa 1922; courtesy of the Minnesota Historical Society

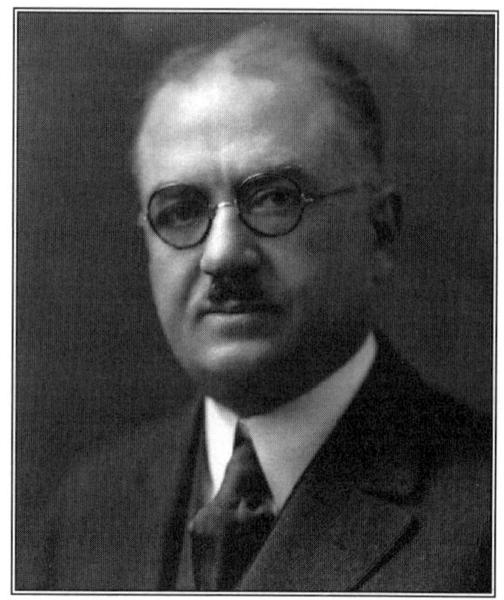

S. (Solon) Marx White, M.D., 1873-1966; Internal Medicine
Photo circa 1921; courtesy of the Minnesota Historical Society

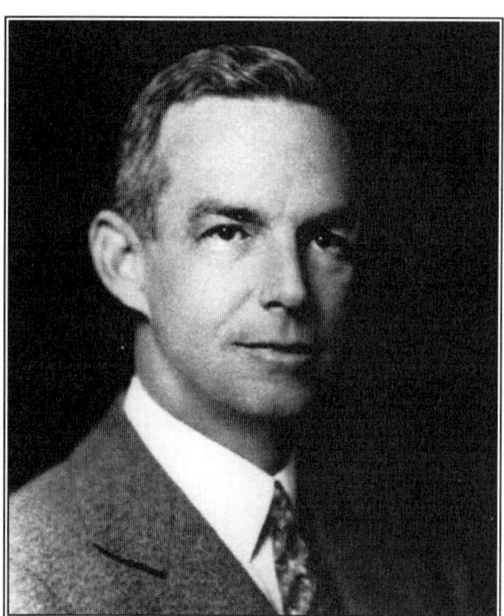

Angus Washburn Morrison, M.D., 1883-1948; Neuropsychiatry
Photo circa 1933; courtesy of the University of Minnesota archives

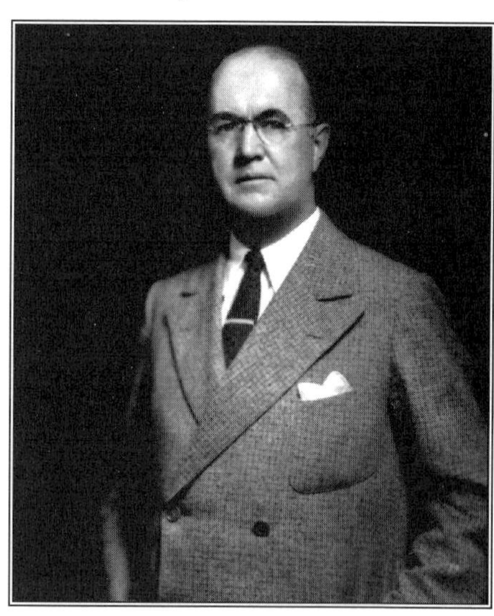

Gilbert Joshua Thomas, M.D., 1884-1969; Urology
Photo circa 1937; Kaiden Keystone Photos, courtesy of the Minnesota Historical Society

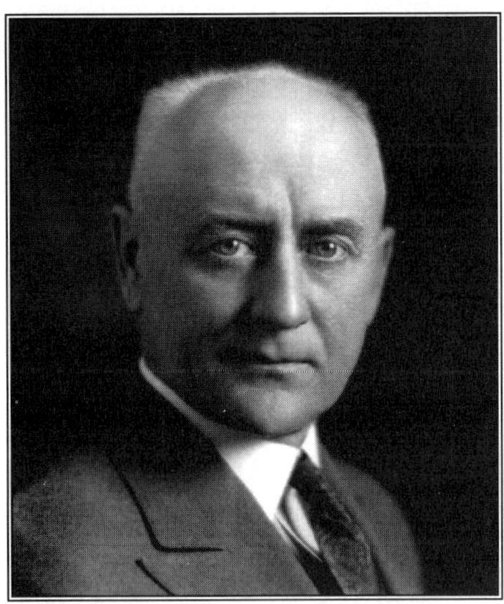

James Andrew Johnson, M.D., 1883–1974;
Surgery
Photo circa 1936; courtesy of the Northwestern University archives

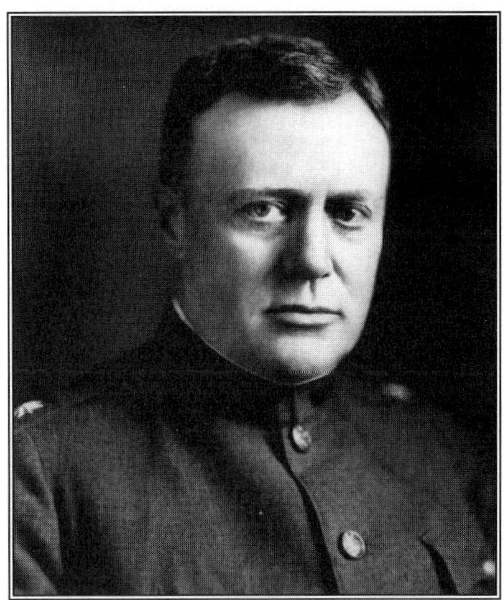

Louis Benedict Baldwin, M.D., 1872–1926;
Business Administration
Photo circa 1918; courtesy of the University of Minnesota archives

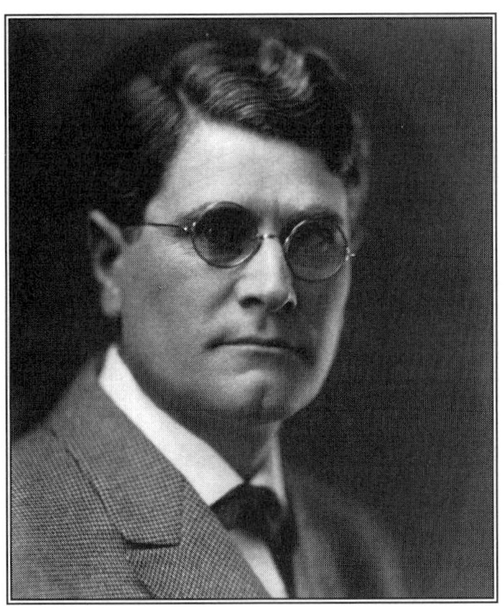

Arthur Clarence Strachauer, M.D., 1883–1957;
Surgery
Photo circa 1922; courtesy of the University of Minnesota archives

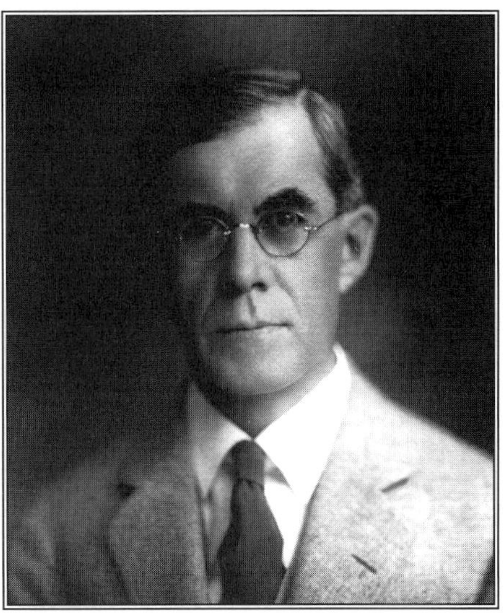

William Robbins Murray, M.D., 1869–1926;
Eye, Ear, Nose, Throat
Photo circa 1923; courtesy of the University of Minnesota archives

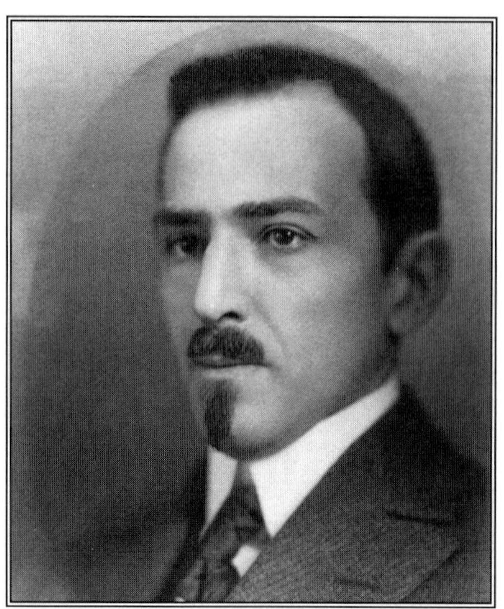

John Peter Schneider, M.D., 1879–1950; Internal Medicine
Photo circa 1921; courtesy of the University of Minnesota archives

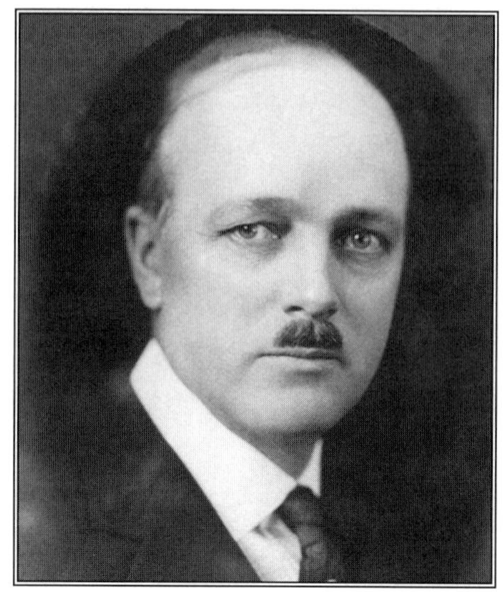

Charles Anthony Reed, M.D., 1872–1950; Orthopedics
Photo circa 1922; courtesy of the University of Minnesota archives

ASSOCIATES

JAMES B. CAREY, M.D.; INTERNAL MEDICINE
WILLIAM H. CONDIT, M.D.; OBSTETRICS AND GYNECOLOGY
OLGA S. HANSEN, M.D.; INTERNAL MEDICINE
MANLEY H. HAYNES, M.D.; OBSTETRICS AND GYNECOLOGY
EVERETT E. MACGIBBON, D.D.S.; DENTISTRY
F. H. K. SCHAAF, M.D.; INTERNAL MEDICINE

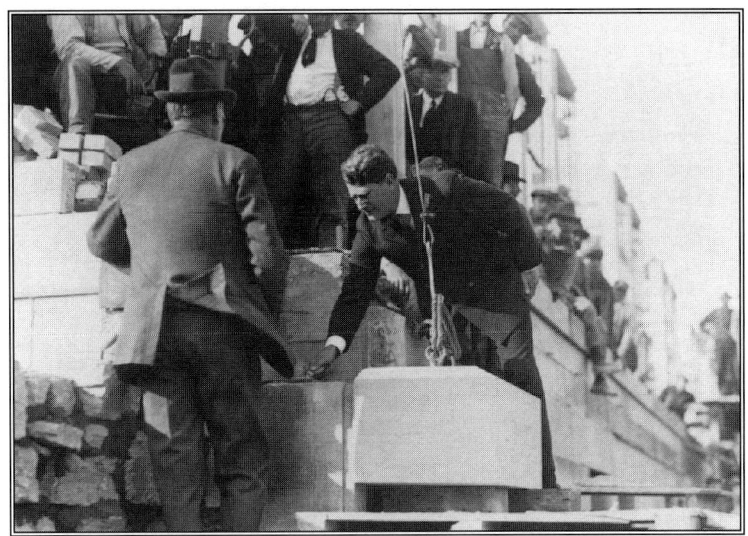

Dr. Arthur C. Strachauer, cofounder of the Nicollet Clinic and chief of the university's department of surgery from 1919–1925, laying the cornerstone of George Chase Christian Memorial Cancer Hospital, University of Minnesota. Photo circa 1924; courtesy of the Minnesota Historical Society

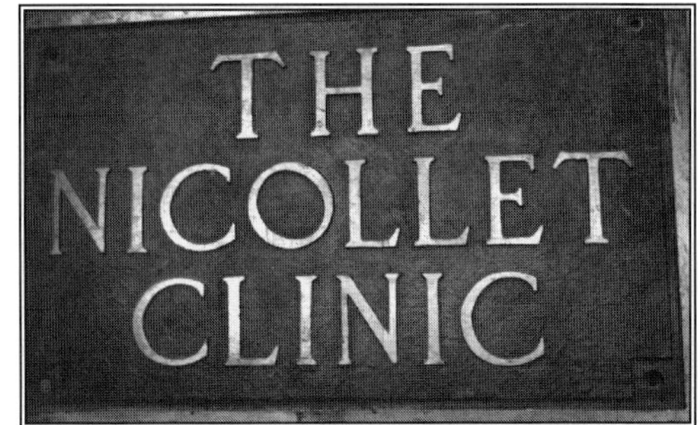

Nameplate from original building

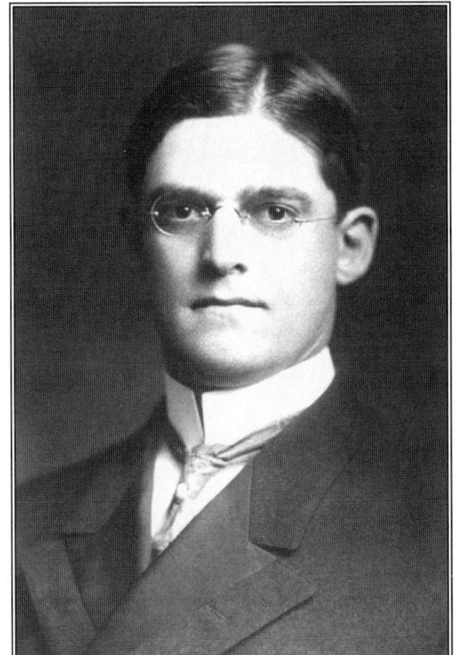

Dr. William Henry Condit, obstetrician at the Nicollet Clinic from 1921 to 1952. Photo circa 1912; courtesy of the University of Minnesota archives

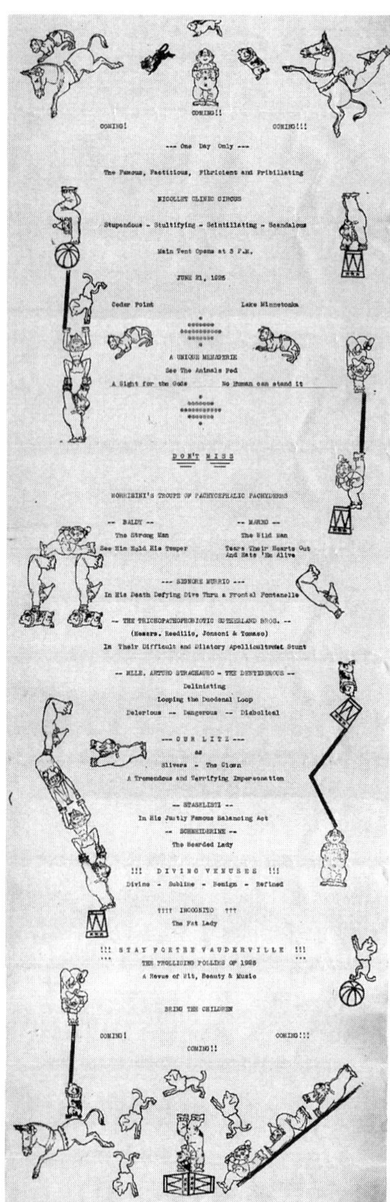

COMING!!

COMING! COMING!!!

--- One Day Only ---

The Famous, Factitious, Fibricient and Fribillating

NICOLLET CLINIC CIRCUS

Stupendous - Stultifying - Scintillating - Scandalous

Main Tent Opens at 3 P.M.

JUNE 21, 1925

Cedar Point Lake Minnetonka

A UNIQUE MENAGERIE

See The Animals Fed

A Sight for the Gods No Human can stand it

DON'T MISS

MORRISINI'S TROUPE OF PACHYCEPHALIC PACHYDERMS

-- BALDY --
The Strong Man
See Him Hold His Temper

-- MARKO --
The Wild Man
Tears Their Hearts Out
And Eats 'Em Alive

--- SIGNORE MURRIO ---
In His Death Defying Dive Thru a Frontal Fontanelle

-- THE TRICHOPATHOPHOBIOTIC SUTHERLAND BROS. --
(Messrs. Reedilio, Jonsoni & Tomaso)
In Their Difficult and Dilatory Apellicultredet Stunt

-- MLLE. ARTURO STRACHAURO - THE DENTIDEROUS --
Delinisting
Looping the Duodenal Loop
Delerious -- Dangerous -- Diabolical

--- O U R L I T Z ---
as
Slivers - The Clown
A Tremendous and Terrifying Impersonation

-- STASELISTI --
In His Justly Famous Balancing Act
-- SCHNEIDERINE --
The Bearded Lady

!!! D I V I N G V E N U S E S !!!
Divine - Sublime - Benign - Refined

???? INCOGNITO ???
The Fat Lady

!!! S T A Y F O R T H E V A U D E R V I L L E !!!
THE FROLLICING FOLLIES OF 1925
A Revue of Wit, Beauty & Music

BRING THE CHILDREN

COMING! COMING!!!

COMING!!

An invitation to the Nicollet Clinic annual picnic, circa 1925

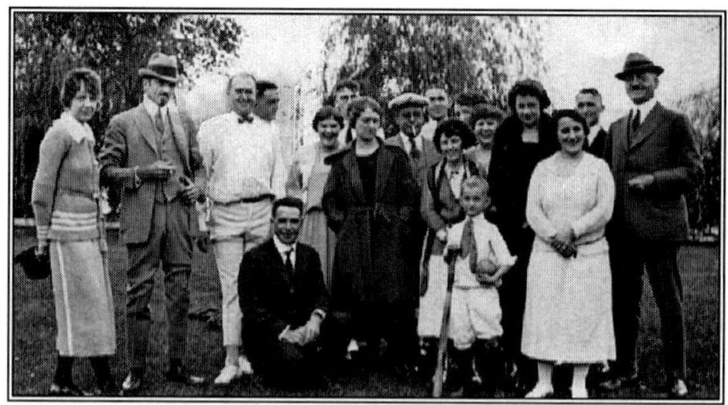

The Nicollet Clinic staff celebrates the fifteenth anniversary, circa 1936

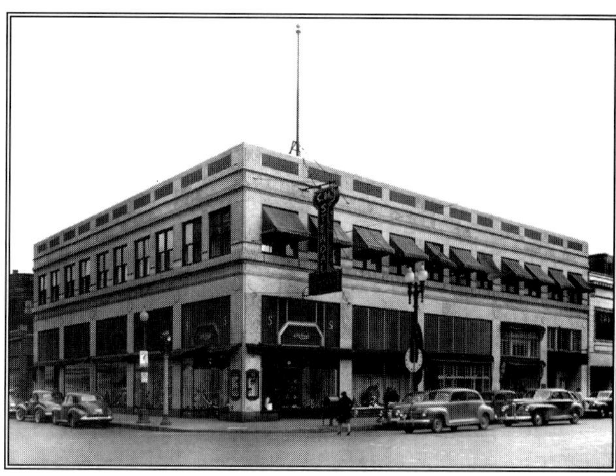

The Nicollet Clinic opened January 25, 1921 in the second story of this building at 1009 Nicollet Avenue, Minneapolis.
Photo circa 1947; Norton & Peel Photography

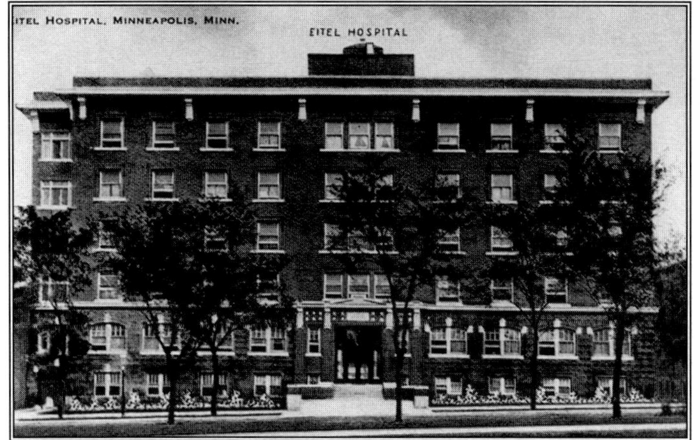

The Nicollet Clinic purchased Eitel Hospital at 1375 Willow Street in the spring of 1929. In 1957 the hospital established a lay board of leaders and changed from a private to a community hospital. The Nicollet Clinic and Eitel Hospital maintained a spirit of close collaboration for another twenty-five years. Photo (postcard) circa 1914; courtesy of the Minnesota Historical Society

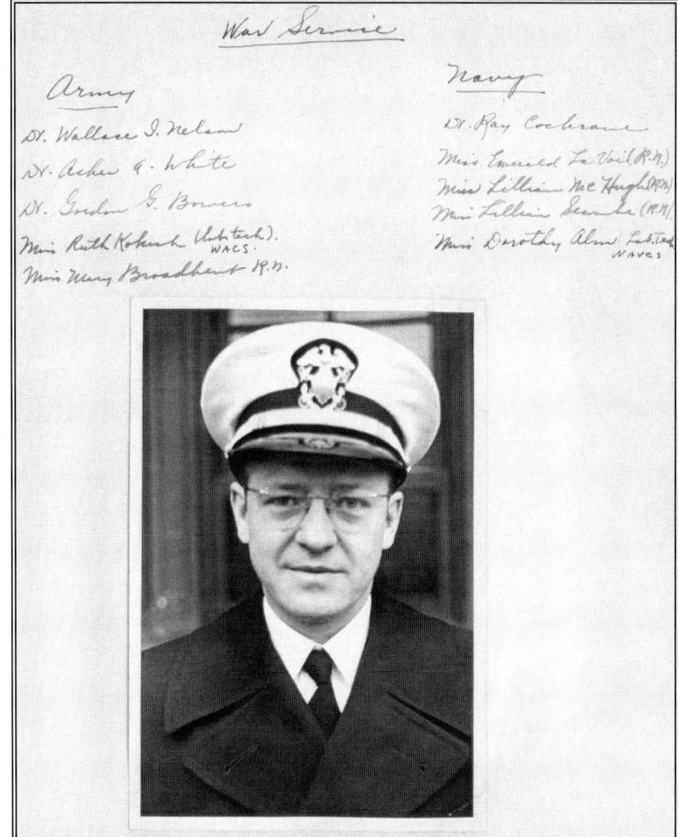

War Service

Army

Dr. Wallace I. Nelson
Dr. Archie G. White
Dr. Gordon G. Bowers
Miss Ruth Kohrsh (lab tech.) WACS
Miss Mary Broadbent R.N.

Navy

Dr. Ray Cochrane
Miss Emerald La Voil (R.N.)
Miss Lillian McHugh (R.N.)
Miss Lillian [illegible] (R.N.)
Miss Dorothy Alm Lab. Tech. NAVES

This page from the Nicollet Clinic scrapbook notes those staff members serving in World War II, circa 1941. Photo of Dr. Ray Cochrane.

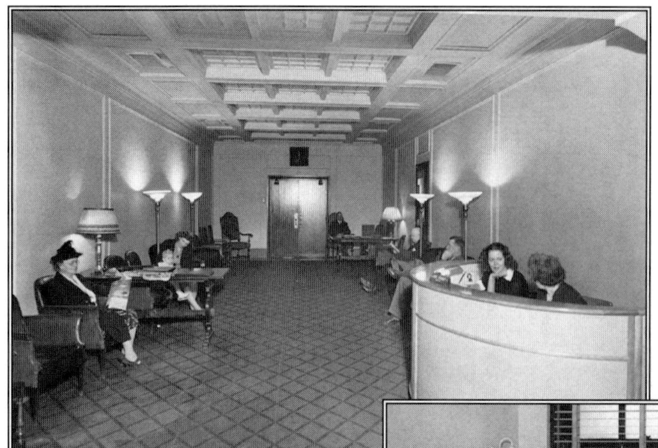

The Nicollet Clinic lobby at 1009 Nicollet Avenue, Minneapolis
Photo circa 1947; Norton & Peel Photography

Dr. S. Marx White at 1009 Nicollet Avenue, Minneapolis
Photo circa 1947; Norton & Peel Photography

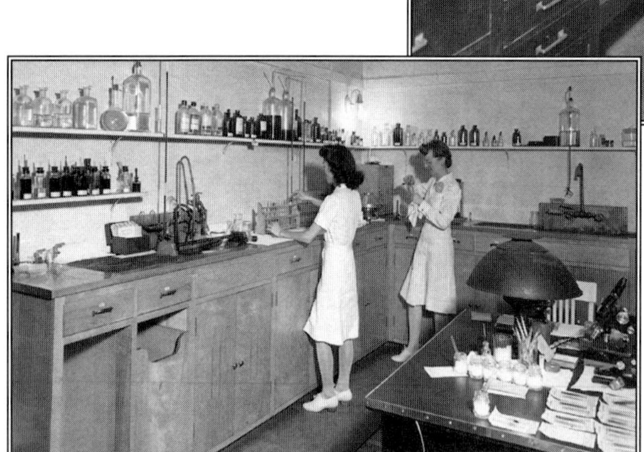

The Nicollet Clinic laboratory at 1009 Nicollet Avenue, Minneapolis
Photo circa 1947; Norton & Peel Photography

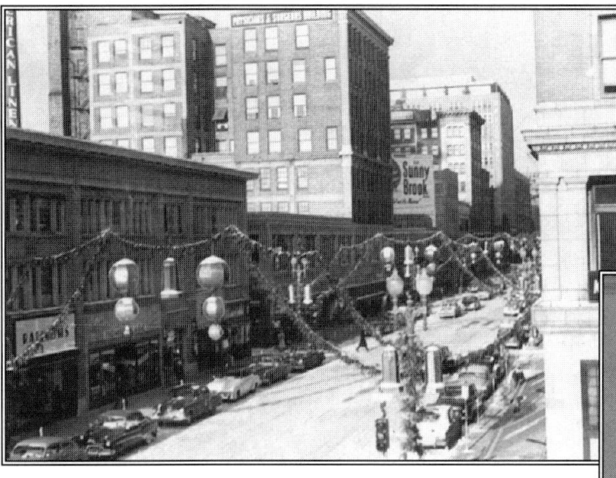

Nicollet Avenue decorated for Christmas, circa 1951

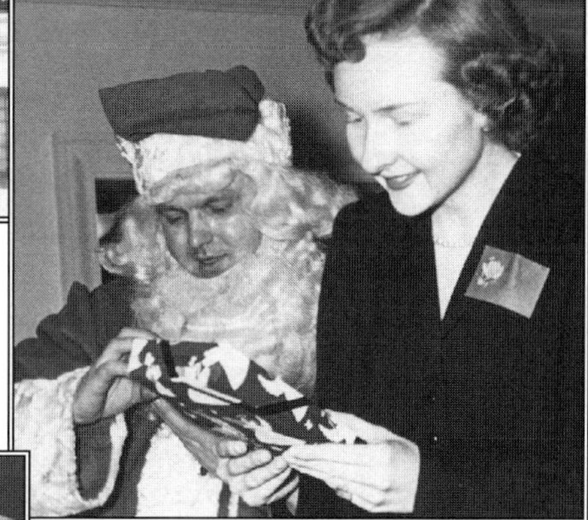

Robert L. Newell and Ruth Kuhlman

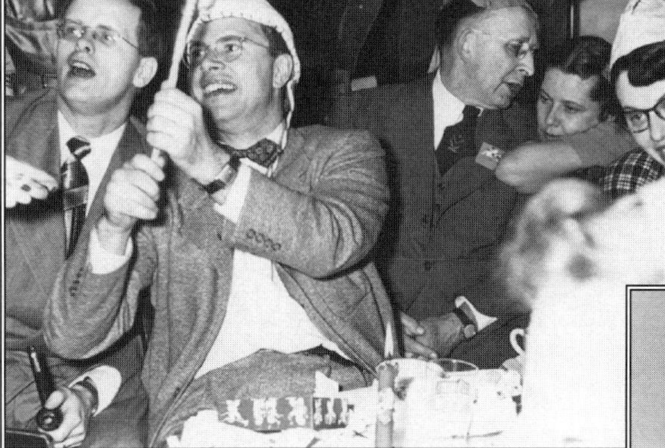

Drs. Fred Rice, Wallace Lueck, and Hugo Altnow; Dorothy Gale, and Donna Reiehmuth

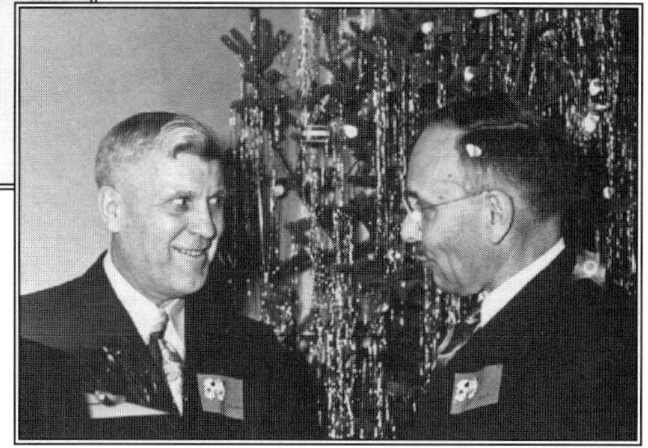

Ray Rainbolt (left) and Dr. Melvin Baken, Sr.

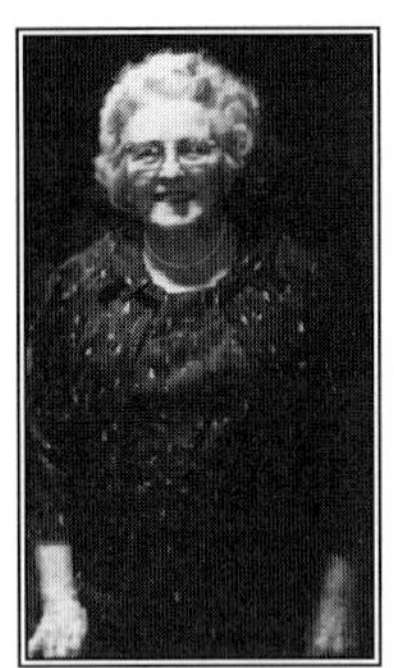

Gertrude Stewart, "Skeeter," registrar and assistant personnel director at the Nicollet Clinic from 1921–1965. Miss Stewart's careful compilation of two scrapbooks proved invaluable in the development of this book.

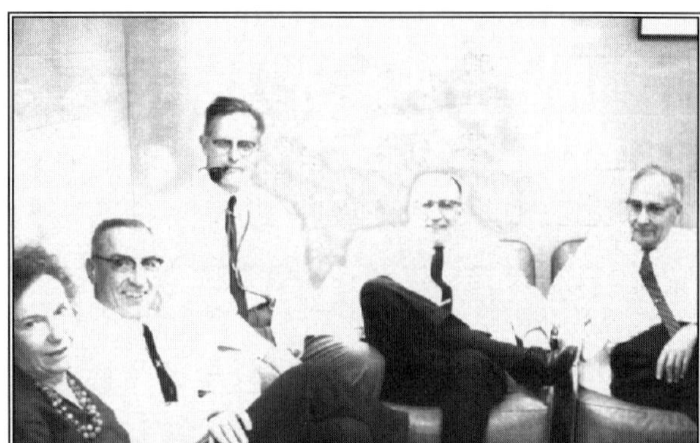

Drs. Olga Hansen, Asher White, Fred Rice, Robert Cranston, and Melvin Baken, Sr. at 1963 Christmas party.

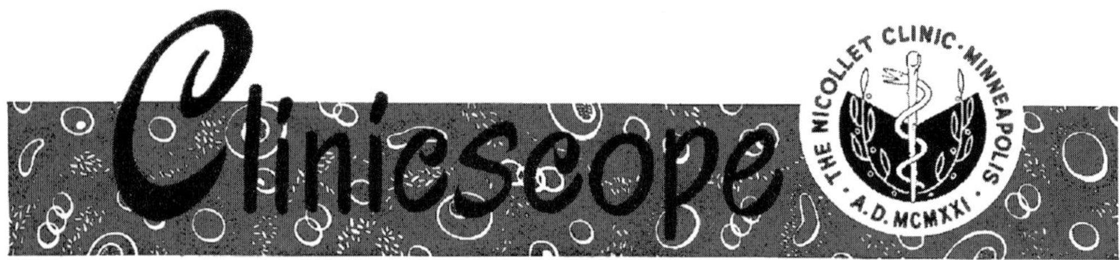

Cliniscope newsletter masthead circa 1953

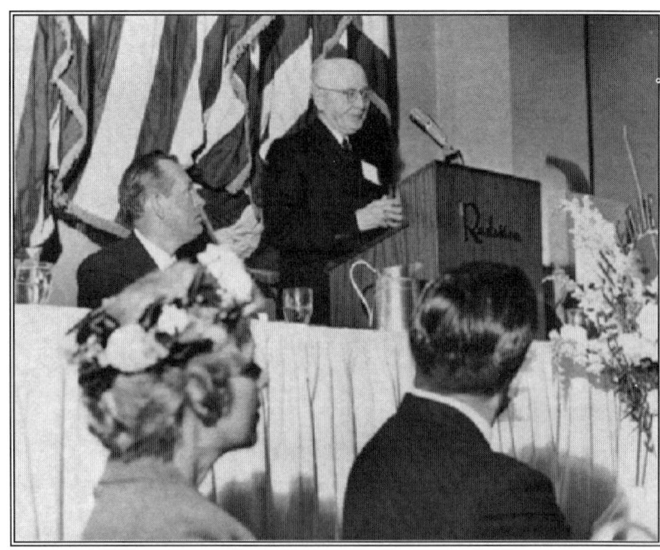

Dr. James A. Johnson is honored by the American Cancer Society for his years of devotion and service. Photo circa 1959 courtesy of the American Cancer Society

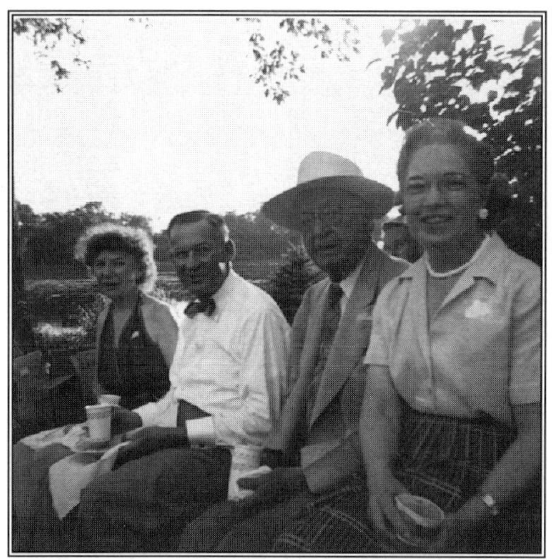

Drs. Olga Hansen, Wallace Nelson, S. Marx White; and Viola Quast, R.N.

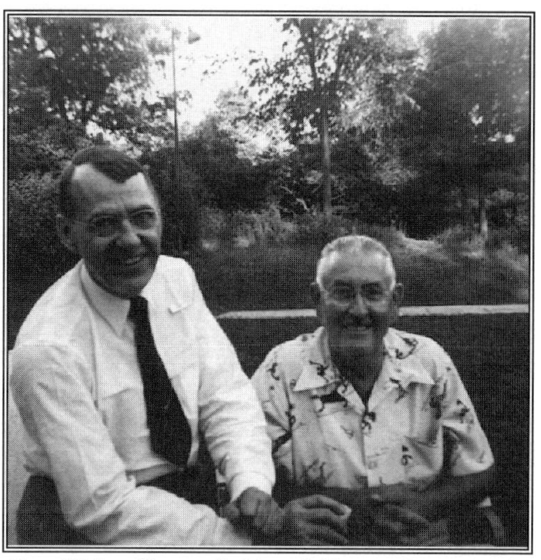

Drs. Walter Haven (left) and Clayton Swanson, Sr.

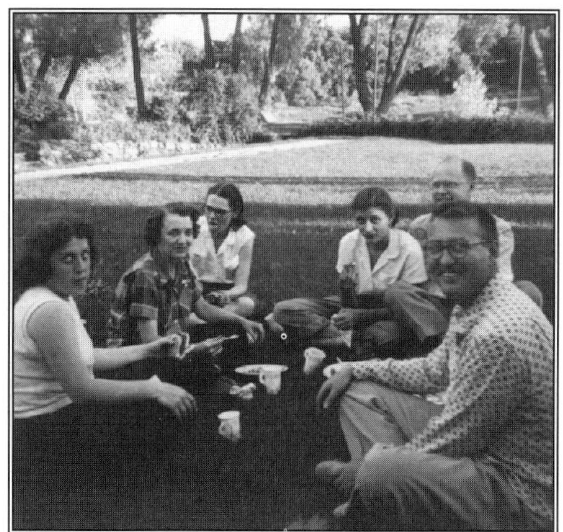

Family and friends

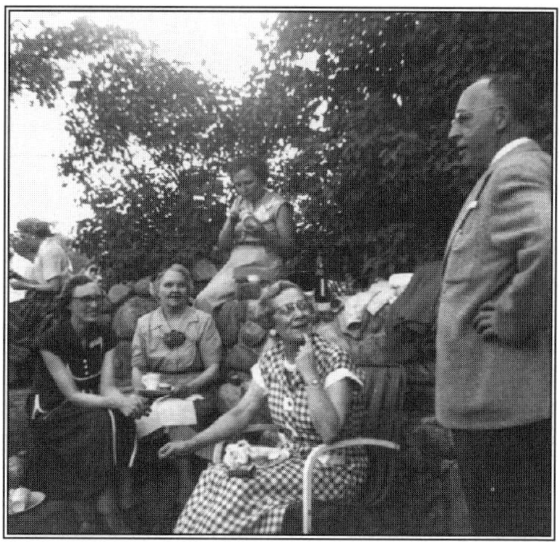

Ardel Lande, Ida B. Johnson (bookkeeper), Alice Hanson (switchboard), and Dr. Hugo Altnow

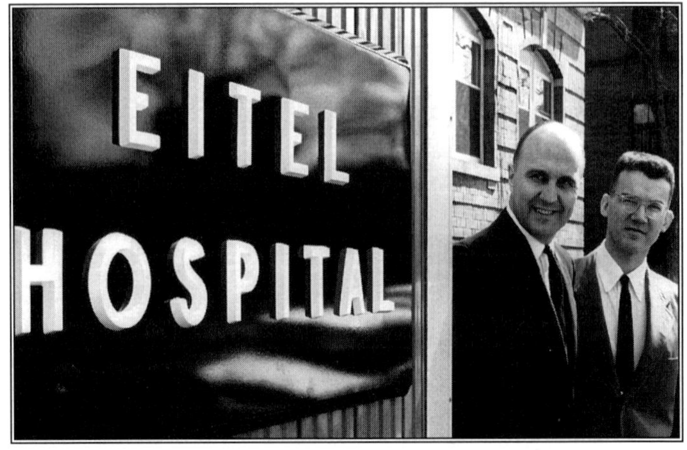

Named for Dr. George Eitel, a nationally prominent surgeon, Eitel Hospital was renamed "Doctors Memorial Hospital" in 1954 to honor the many physicians who helped build its reputation. Because this confused the public, in 1960 the name was changed back to Eitel Hospital. Looking at the new sign are Jack Rivall (left), hospital adminstrator, and Dr. Arthur Ide, Jr., chief of staff. Photo © 1996 Star Tribune/Minneapolis-St. Paul

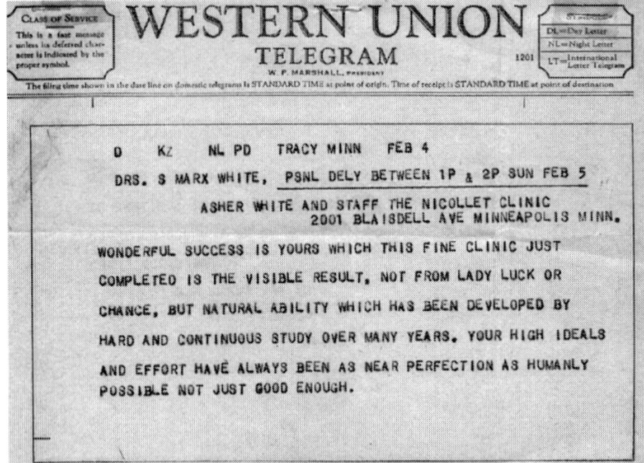

WESTERN UNION
TELEGRAM
W. P. MARSHALL, PRESIDENT

D KZ NL PD TRACY MINN FEB 4
DRS. S MARX WHITE, PSNL DELY BETWEEN 1P & 2P SUN FEB 5
ASHER WHITE AND STAFF THE NICOLLET CLINIC
2001 BLAISDELL AVE MINNEAPOLIS MINN.

WONDERFUL SUCCESS IS YOURS WHICH THIS FINE CLINIC JUST COMPLETED IS THE VISIBLE RESULT, NOT FROM LADY LUCK OR CHANCE, BUT NATURAL ABILITY WHICH HAS BEEN DEVELOPED BY HARD AND CONTINUOUS STUDY OVER MANY YEARS. YOUR HIGH IDEALS AND EFFORT HAVE ALWAYS BEEN AS NEAR PERFECTION AS HUMANLY POSSIBLE NOT JUST GOOD ENOUGH.

THE COMPANY WILL APPRECIATE SUGGESTIONS FROM ITS PATRONS CONCERNING ITS SERVICE

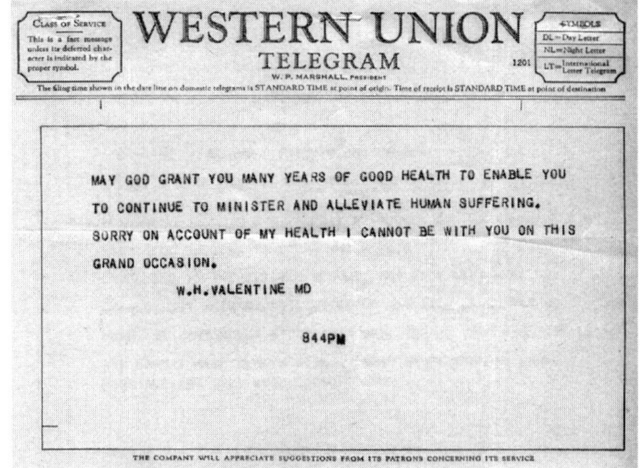

WESTERN UNION
TELEGRAM
W. P. MARSHALL, PRESIDENT

MAY GOD GRANT YOU MANY YEARS OF GOOD HEALTH TO ENABLE YOU TO CONTINUE TO MINISTER AND ALLEVIATE HUMAN SUFFERING. SORRY ON ACCOUNT OF MY HEALTH I CANNOT BE WITH YOU ON THIS GRAND OCCASION.

W.H.VALENTINE MD

844PM

THE COMPANY WILL APPRECIATE SUGGESTIONS FROM ITS PATRONS CONCERNING ITS SERVICE

Congratulatory telegram received at the Nicollet Clinic open house celebration, February 5, 1961.

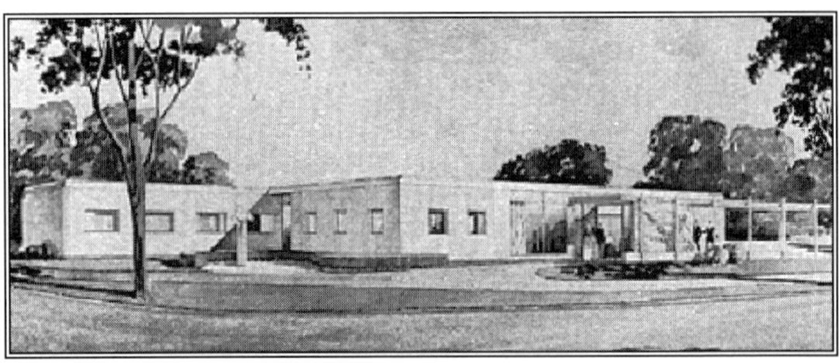

The Nicollet Clinic moved to a new facility at 2001 Blaisdell Avenue, Minneapolis, on September 26, 1960. Illustration by Ellerbe and Associates

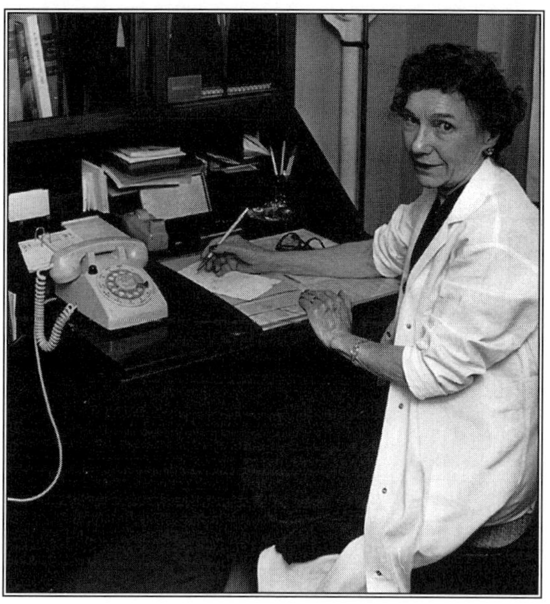

Dr. Olga S. Hansen is recognized for fifty years in medicine in a newspaper article on June 6, 1965.
Photo © 1996 StarTribune/Minneapolis-St. Paul

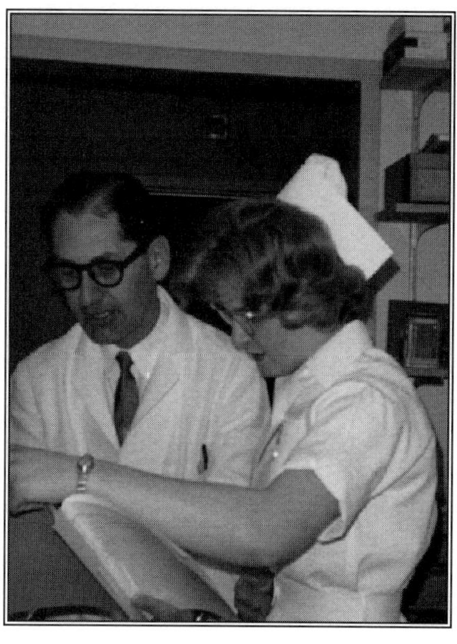

Pediatrician Theodore C. Papermaster and Marlene Wilson, R.N., circa 1965

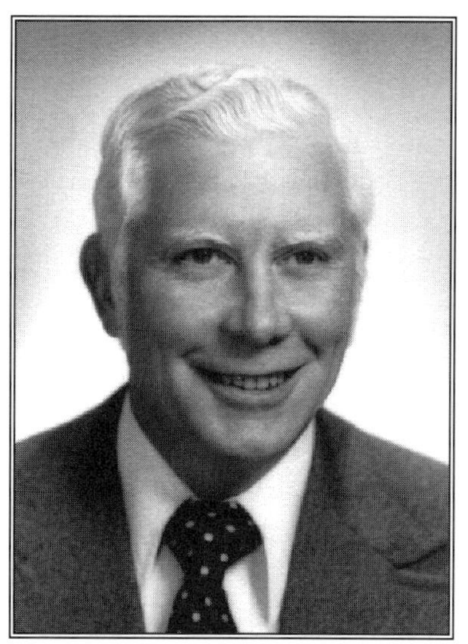

William Costello, business manager at the Nicollet Clinic from 1962 to 1983

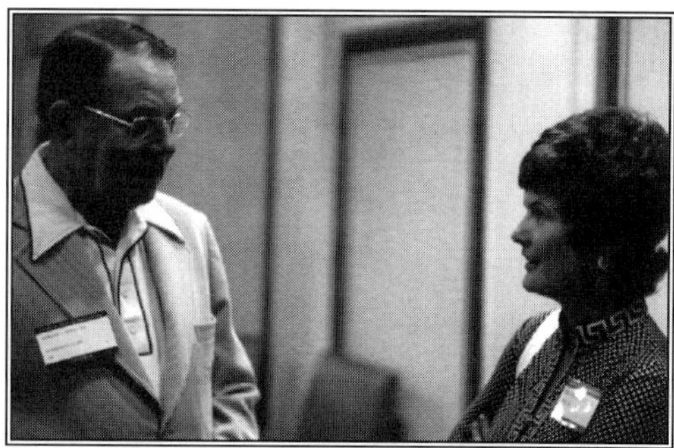

Dr. Howard Horns and Mrs. William (Dorothy) Costello at an American Medical Association meeting in June, 1974.

The Nicollet Clinic
wishes to announce the opening of a suburban office
at 6630 Lyndale Avenue South, Richfield
for Northrop Beach, M. D.
of the Department of Pediatrics

Hours by appointment at the Nicollet Clinic or	6630 Lyndale Avenue South Main 3411

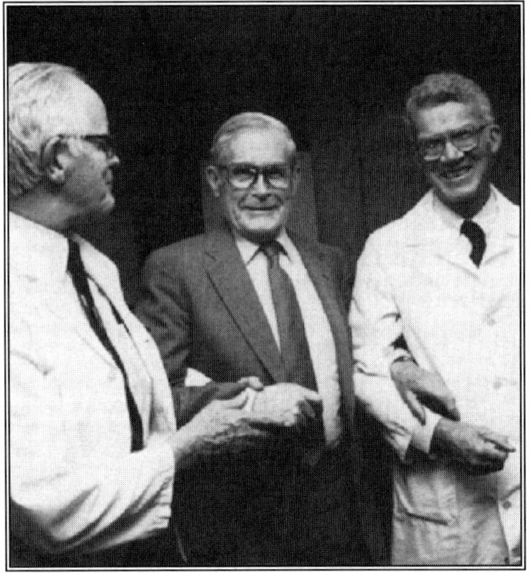

In 1950, at a time when most medical practices were in downtown Minneapolis, pediatrician Northrop Beach opened a branch of the Nicollet Clinic pediatrics department in the suburb of Richfield. Run by pediatric nurse Ruth Erickson and staffed by Dr. Beach, the pioneering satellite clinic served patients from the Richfield, Bloomington, and Pilot Knob areas.

In 1986 the "Northrop Beach, M.D. Pediatric Wing" was dedicated at the 2001 Blaisdell Avenue clinic site in honor of his longstanding association with the Nicollet Clinic. Giving warm regards to Beach (center) are Drs. Fred Rice (left) and Arthur Ide.

Part Two
St. Louis Park Medical Center

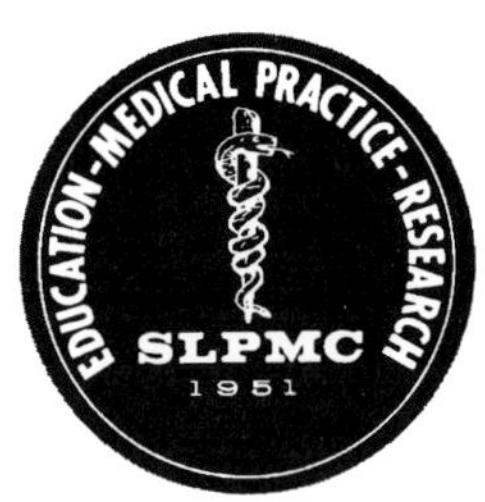

6

REINVENTING GROUP PRACTICE
THE FOUNDING OF ST. LOUIS PARK MEDICAL CENTER

In the fall of 1949, four years after the end of World War II, a news article caught the attention of a young surgeon nearing the end of his surgical residency in the University of Minnesota Medical School. The article, prominently placed on the business page of the *Minneapolis Star* and complete with an architect's rendering, described a proposed new medical office building in the Minneapolis suburb of St. Louis Park.[1]

The surgeon, Richard J. Webber, seized on the intended development as a possible solution to a puzzle that he had been working on: How does one go about starting a medical practice in an underserved area with no capital, no patients, and no practice history? At a time when the vast majority of medical specialists practiced as individuals in downtown Minneapolis, where would he find financial support for his doubly unorthodox idea to create a multispecialty group practice in the suburbs?

Webber had been conducting his own informal survey of the suburban ring, and had already settled on St. Louis Park as a potential location for an office. Discovering a developer who had already identified the need for medical services in the suburbs was enough to convince Webber to move ahead. He called to set up an initial meeting with the developer and, with that call, started a process that would change the face of medicine in Minneapolis.

As Webber prepared for his meeting with Nicholas Phillips, the developer, he studied the description of the planned office building and became more and more excited. "If there was to be a group of offices," Webber thought, "why wouldn't it be reasonable to offer to staff [the offices] with a group of well-trained specialists in various fields of medical practice?"[2] Webber had early on rejected the option of creating a surgical specialty group in the suburbs. He was certain, based on his experience as a battalion surgeon in the Pacific theater during the war and on his observations of his father's medical practice at the Duluth West Side Clinic, that a multispecialty group offered significant benefits to the physician and to the patient. Not the least of these potential benefits was the time away from day-to-day practice a group clinic could afford its individual specialists interested in retaining an active role in medical research and education.

Webber resolved to take this idea to Phillips. They met at the Lilac Way Shopping Center, the site of the proposed medical offices, which was strategically located at the corner of Route 100 and Excelsior Boulevard. After talking with Phillips, Webber went home convinced that his idea of establishing a multispecialty group in St. Louis Park had a strong ally. With Phillips' support, his idea moved from the realm of the pipe dream to something more tangible. Webber was ready to introduce the idea to his colleagues.

RECRUITING THE GROUP

Webber, who was just thirty-two at the time, took his plans to two of his friends and contemporaries at the Veterans Administration Hospital, David M. Anderson, a urologist, and Robert R. Geibink, an orthopedist. Like Webber,

Anderson and Geibink were finishing their residencies and thinking of the future. Both shared Webber's interest in developing the ideal group practice and quickly signed on to the project.

At the center of this ideal group would be internal medicine, the keystone of the organization and its largest department. To pull this department together, Webber next called on Robert A. (Bud) Green, then thirty-two and an instructor of internal medicine at the University of Minnesota. "We had been good friends in medical school," Green recalled in 1994, "and I had a lot of respect for his judgment. Cecil Watson, our department chair, was pushing me toward basic research and I knew that wasn't my forte. But the prospect of combining patient care, teaching, and clinical research with a group of my own choosing really caught fire inside of me. I didn't hesitate a minute."

Green took his job to heart and easily recruited John W. LaBree and Wyman E. Jacobson, who were, like himself, chief residents at the end of their specialty training. Each man had been struggling with the same decision Green had: academic medicine or private practice? When the opportunity came to perhaps have the best of both, the choice was easy.

Recalling his time as a resident, LaBree said, "Bud and I had been looking for something to do. We would get together on weekends with our wives and debate whether or not we would go into private practice or remain academics . . . but we hadn't really done anything about it. So when this thing hit, it was just a catalyst. Suddenly, we knew that this was the thing to do." Jacobson, who knew Green only by name and reputation, said he was "a little taken aback" by the call, but added, "I was thrilled to get the invitation. I had been planning to stay in academic medicine, but it didn't take long before I called back with a yes."

With this group of six quickly and enthusiastically assembled, regular planning meetings began to take place at the University Campus Club. Each physician put $125 into the treasury to cover organizing expenses, and they went to work.

Green and LaBree continued the job of recruiting. By January 1950, they added Alex Barno and Donald W. Freeman to the group to create the obstetrics and gynecology department. Both had worked closely with Professor John L. McKelvey, chair of the university's Department of Obstetrics and Gynecology, in developing the Minnesota Maternal Mortality Study, continuing the pioneering work of Jennings C. Litzenberg in the first half of the century.

By the spring of 1950, the initial roster of specialists was complete with the addition of Sewell S. Gordon, a radiologist, and Arnold S. Anderson, a pediatrician. Pediatrics was felt to be an especially important area for the group. St. Louis Park was growing rapidly. Its population of 7,700 in 1940 had almost tripled to 23,000 in 1950. There were "more preschool age children in the Park waiting to enter school," the St. Louis Park Dispatch wrote in October 1949, "than are already enrolled in the twelve grades of the school system."[3] Anderson, a pediatric fellow at the Mayo Foundation's Growth and Development Institute, had the experience and dedication to handle what was sure to be a large part of the practice. In the fall of 1950, Anderson recruited George W. Lund to join him, and Lund became the eleventh and final member of the founding partnership.

CRISIS TO OPPORTUNITY

While Green and LaBree were working on recruitment, Webber, Geibink, and Jacobson were trying to nail down an agreement with the developer, Nick Phillips. The planning was going slowly. Engineering problems had been encountered in renovating the Lilac Way Shopping Center, but the group persisted. They persisted because they could see no alternative and because the shopping center was so ideally situated on the corner of one of the busiest intersections in the state. Lilac Way promised the new clinic high visibility in St. Louis Park, and easy access from anywhere in the western half of the metropolitan area.[4] As problems surfaced, solutions were found, according to Wyman Jacobson, creating "the greatest sense of group solidarity you can imagine."

Late in 1949, the time came to finalize a contract with Phillips. Gathered together and ready to leap collectively into their future, the group found themselves staring into an abyss of unfavorable terms, costs, and conditions. The group caucused, hoping to find some way to recover their momentum. Dr. Richard Varco, a friend from the University of Minnesota who had been attending some of the group's meetings, put words to a heretofore unimaginable thought: Why not build the clinic themselves?[5] At this suggestion, defeat metamorphosed into excitement. The shock of the sudden collapse of the Lilac Way negotiations served to harden the group's resolve to control their own destiny. They would develop their own space.

ASSISTANCE ARRIVES

With more determination than good sense the group moved ahead, continuing to meet on a weekly basis. The obstacles seemed almost insurmountable. They had no site, no building, no source of financing, and no established practices to impress a banker.

At a meeting on February 1, 1950, Robert Geibink reported that he had contacted the owners of a small nursery and garden center on the corner of Excelsior Boulevard and Quentin Avenue, who had agreed to consider leasing a portion of the nursery property. The owners, Morten and Katheren Arneson, returned to St. Louis Park from their

Remembering the sale of his land to the young physicians Arneson wrote, "I had to swallow a few bad-tasting pills, because the financial arrangement was rather one-sided, but I was happy about it and it gave me great pleasure to follow [the medical center's] progress."[7] Eleven years later, on the occasion of dedicating the clinic library to the Arnesons, Richard Webber tried to capture the group's strong affection for their benefactors. "Our request for your property," Webber said, "was foolish. You were using the land for your own nursery enterprise. The terms we could offer were limited. How wonderful that you were interested! You became an agent for our welfare and success. The clinic survived because of your faith in it. It succeeded because you and Katheren became its godparents and provided us a chance to meet opportunity."[8]

Florida winter home, where Geibink had contacted them, in late February to prepare for the spring nursery season. "For some reason," Morten Arneson wrote later, "the request . . . had definite appeal to me," though he had previously rejected numerous offers for his land. Several days after arriving back in St. Louis Park, Arneson was, by his own account, in bed with a bad cold when the doorbell announced the arrival, en masse, of the protean medical group. Wedged into his small front room, Arneson recalled, was "this group of fine-looking young doctors, clean-cut, intelligent, and desirous of forming a partnership." Listening to the story of their search for a place to build a medical center, Arneson felt his defensive mood disappear: "I became eager to have them locate on my land. . . . I felt with men like that working together, the clinic could not help but be a great success."[6]

At that meeting the Arnesons made their first of many contributions to the group, agreeing to lease the western portion of their three-acre nursery, a portion with 100 feet of frontage on Excelsior Boulevard, for a below-market price within the limited means of the young physicians. The lease of $1,000 per year—with a ten-year option to buy the parcel for $20,000—was made even more affordable by the Arnesons' willingness to allow the first payment to be delayed until the building was occupied.

SEEKING CAPITAL

The group now had a location on the map to which they could pin their hopes. With new energy, they continued the search for financing, for architectural and management advice, and for a contractor willing to commit to the project. The group prepared a prospectus and divided up the task of visiting each of the commercial banks in Minneapolis. After almost a month of meetings, none of the banks had expressed an interest in the young group, and none were willing to extend financing.

Finally, in March 1950, a local banker with an interest in the needs of his growing community identified a creative solution. Gerald P. Utley of Minnesota Federal Savings and Loan, St. Louis Park branch, suggested that the physicians, all veterans, pool their unused GI housing loan guarantees. If the Veterans Administration approved pooling the benefits, Utley told the group, Minnesota Federal would risk $50,000 on the project, and up to another $50,000 guaranteed by the GI Bill.

With the promise of financing, the group spent the summer creating a legal partnership, completing the financial paperwork needed to fulfill the loan application requirements, and designing their new building. Many hours were spent at the University Campus Club, debating practice procedures and developing minimum space and equipment requirements for each department. Robert Cerny of Long and Thorshov Architects, a friend and neighbor of John LaBree's, completed the building design. The L-shaped plan featured a sunny, glass entryway and waiting area facing Excelsior Boulevard, twenty examining rooms, a surgery suite, fifteen offices, a laboratory, and a radiology suite, all of which promised to satisfy the group's desire for a functional and attractive workplace. Its major drawback, the lack of expansion space, would become painfully obvious in only a few years.

In early August 1950, Carl E. Lebeck and Company was selected as general contractor for the new St. Louis Park Medical Center with a low bid of $124,380. Because strikes in the mining and steel industries and the growing conflict in Korea were creating nationwide materials shortages and rapidly escalating costs, the construction contract included a cost-escalator clause if the project start was delayed beyond August 15. The loan had to be approved by the deadline, if construction were to remain within the price of the bid.

On August 15, the day the fixed-price contract would expire, Wyman Jacobson was attending a seminar in

Washington, D.C.[9] Realizing that he was only a few blocks from the Veterans Administration loan guarantee offices, Jacobson took it upon himself to see what could be done. He soon found himself sitting before a young loan officer in charge of small-business loans. While waiting for the man to finish a phone call, Jacobson noticed his own loan application on the very top of a stack of forms. "I told the man who I was and that I wanted to see what could be done about this application on his desk," Jacobson remembered. "He told me he was ready to approve it, but was going to call the next week to get answers to some questions he had." Jacobson answered the questions on the spot. "I saw him take the stamp and mark it approved," a development Jacobson still considers "the best stroke of luck I ever had."

With only hours before the fixed-price contract expired, Jacobson wired the news of the Veterans Administration approval to Richard Webber, who called a special meeting. With the wire message in hand, the entire group jumped in their cars and raced over to Carl Lebeck's home. Roused from sleep at 11:00 p.m., Lebeck heard the news that the loans had been approved and, with some persuading, agreed to honor his contract.

Gerald Utley was true to his word also. Minnesota Federal sent the final notice of approval on August 24, 1950. The $96,000 loan at 4 percent, of which $36,000 was guaranteed by the Veterans Administration, required the group to raise the remaining $30,000. By September, the ten partners (George Lund was not yet part of the group) had each raised $3,500, a major feat for men who had been living on relatively meager academic and military salaries.

A PHILOSOPHY OF PRACTICE

During the long wait for the building to be finished, the group had time to debate and refine their practice philosophy.

Central to their philosophy were the ideals of multispecialty group practice. As Jacobson put it in 1952, group practice "offers the best chance for reasonable economic stability and individual security with the least compromise of basic medical principles and self respect." Within the structure of mutual support, it became financially feasible to provide for "time away from medical practice to pursue research, teaching, and other educational activities leading to continued professional growth."[10]

From the beginning, each member of the professional staff was granted one day per week to teach, conduct research, or become involved in other community work approved by the group. In 1952, two years after the group in St. Louis Park had written explicit support for research and education into their partnership bylaws, the Truman Commission on the Health Needs of the Nation lauded group practice as a "characteristically American response to the need for organization of health services . . . an important answer to the problems which are posed by the increasing complexity of medical science and technology. Physicians working together in a group," the report concluded, "continue the best features of their training period throughout their professional lives—the stimulation to keep up with medical progress through constant appraisal by informed colleagues and ready access to consultation and technical assistance."[11] St. Louis Park Medical Center was dedicated to taking this one step further by retaining ties to the University of Minnesota while developing clinical research programs of its own, thus supporting the continuous refinement of the skills and specialization of its medical staff.

"I am certain," Wyman Jacobson said in his chief-of-staff address to his colleagues in 1952, "that in this present group of varied personalities there is a remarkably unified belief in certain basic ideals. These . . . include a sincere concern for the welfare of the patient, a respect for the dignity of mankind, a deference to the rights of other individuals, and a conviction in the nobleness of purpose of the medical profession."[12]

THE FINANCIAL PICTURE

The next challenge was to translate the ideals of the group into a workable professional partnership agreement that would support the group's clinical research, education, and medical practice goals.[13] The original partnership document, signed in July 1950, included several provisions to implement the egalitarian and academic ideals of the group. First, beginning in July 1951, all income of the partners was to accrue to the partnership. Those with academic or staff appointments contributed their personal income to the general fund. In the interim, those starting new practices would receive salary supplements from partnership funds as necessary. Second, up to 20 percent of each member's time was to be devoted to academic teaching, research, or professional education.

Once the clinic was established, the agreement specified that the group's net income would be divided equally, regardless of bookings or production. A study of group practices by G. Halsey Hunt and Marcus Goldstein, published in 1951, found that although more than three-fourths of the 368 group practices in existence in 1946 were partnerships, only seventeen of these groups had a financial arrangement similar to that set up in 1950 by the founders of St. Louis Park Medical Center.[14] While this was a rare, and to some a subversive financial arrangement, it was reminiscent of the idealism of the early partnership years of the Nicollet Clinic.

MEDICAL COMMUNITY REACTION

The new group in St. Louis Park soon began to feel some of the same opposition from within the medical community that the Nicollet Clinic had had to overcome thirty years before. This ranged from the good-humored, conventional wisdom that "if you move to the suburbs you will starve" to a few incidents of active opposition from professional colleagues.[15] "Although there was strong support from colleagues at the university and some in private practice, there was also widespread antagonism to such a group of young 'pinkos' (as we were designated by a leading Minneapolis internist) entering practice in such an audacious fashion," Robert Green wrote in June 1977. "Failure of the venture was enthusiastically, and by some gleefully, predicted."[16]

One source of resistance the group faced during the first years of practice came from the established hospital medical staffs. Seeing a potential threat in a large, energetic, and well-organized group, most refused to accept more than one or two of the physician members of the medical center. Anderson and LaBree were offered staff privileges at Abbott Hospital, for instance, but Green and the group's surgeons were excluded. "This made it very difficult for us to establish an efficient, coordinated hospital practice," Wyman Jacobson explained. Finding hospital appointments became a first order of business.

By another stroke of good luck, a new two-hundred-bed hospital opened in February 1951. Built by the Minneapolis Jewish community with the support of philanthropist Jay Phillips, Mt. Sinai Hospital was the first private hospital in Minneapolis to have a major teaching affiliation with the University of Minnesota.[17] No strangers to discrimination and anxious to acquire the teaching and clinical skills of the St. Louis Park group for their teaching program, the leaders of Mt. Sinai encouraged the members of the medical center to practice in their facility on Chicago Avenue. With hospital access secured, the ability of opponents within the medical profession to obstruct the growth of St. Louis Park Medical Center was severely limited, a result analogous to the purchase of Eitel Hospital by the Nicollet Clinic in 1929.

In the spring of 1955 St. Louis Park Medical Center was organizing itself to handle the expected crowds of people who would be wanting the Salk polio vaccine. The pediatrics department organized a schedule of evening immunization clinics and mailed an informational flyer on the new vaccine to patients. Whole families, grateful for the convenience, came in to get their shots. Unfortunately, some of the powerful independent physicians in the neighborhood viewed the flyers as a violation of the medical profession's sanction against advertising and filed an ethics complaint with the Hennepin County Medical Society.
"We got a call from the society to come down," said George Lund, "so we sent the Executive Committee. They were meeting at the Minneapolis Club, in the fancy dining room. They didn't ask us to sit down, so we just stood. Then they really gave it to us."

The society decided the flyer was "commercially aggressive and misleading in its contents." Conceding that the group "had acted in good faith," the society nevertheless wished to admonish them against future communications of this kind. . . ."18 Although angered by the incident, the group decided to "kill them with kindness" and thereafter sent representatives to all the society's meetings.[19, 20]

Morten Arneson, on the site every day tending to his own nursery business, appointed himself clerk of the works and "hounded the foreman and the architect incessantly. He provided the water, the electricity, the phone, extra planks, and whatnot for free."[24] To save money, the group had elected to leave part of the basement unexcavated. This, according to Alex Barno, "drove [Arneson] to distraction." As the foundation was being completed, Arneson confronted Robert Cerny, the architect. "'Why don't you get the dirt out of there,' he demanded. 'They will need a full basement.' The architect replied, 'Those fellows don't need a basement.' 'How in the hell do you know?' Morten exploded. 'They might need five buildings before all this is over with.'"[25] Barno—recalling this story in 1966 when the medical center was in two buildings and planning a third—called Arneson a "true prognosticator." Arnold Anderson still ranks leaving the dirt in the basement as one of the worst mistakes they made with the original building.

THE DRIVE TOWARD OPENING DAY

After months of planning and negotiating with bankers, contractors, and architects, ground was finally broken for the St. Louis Park Medical Center in late August 1950. However, as fall turned to winter, materials shortages began to test the group's patience. Work was temporarily halted at times for lack of concrete and steel. Yet, ever resourceful, Morten Arneson and other friends called in favors and, each time, made the necessary contacts to keep construction underway.

Although opening day was set for the first week in July 1951, progress on the building crept along throughout the spring. To no one's great surprise the building wasn't completed on time. Even so, the waiting area and five examining rooms were useable. Anxious to put their dream into action, a cleaning crew of partners and spouses spent the last weekend in June cleaning the plaster dust and construction debris from the space. The crew washed windows and scrubbed floors. Drapes, hand sewn by Marion Jacobson and several other wives, were hung, and the welcome mats laid out.

On Monday morning, July 2, 1951, St. Louis Park Medical Center opened for business without fanfare or public notice, as the medical ethics of the day required. On hand for opening day, besides the eleven founding physicians, were Eloise Giguere, office manager; Monica Doran, X-ray technician; Ag Endres, obstetrics and gynecology nurse; Helen Tarnowski, chief nurse; and John C. Fields, business manager.[21]

Time and distance allow the founders to remember the first days with a bit of humor tinged by nostalgia. With the help of their five original employees, the nine available physicians of the St. Louis Park Medical Center (Robert Geibink and David Anderson were still on duty with the Veterans Administration Hospital) saw five patients on the first day and booked $16. Arnold Anderson saw three of the patients, and Dick Webber saw the other two. "The rest of us just twiddled our thumbs," Alex Barno related fifteen years later. "The first registered patient was Gail Green, two months old and the daughter of Bud and Betty. She was treated for an ear infection at no charge. It took twelve working days to see the first one hundred patients," Barno said. "Fifty-nine of these were seen by pediatrics, twenty-three by medicine, seven by surgery, and five by ob/gyn."[22]

St. Louis Park Medical Center beat the odds assigned by conventional wisdom. The founders had created an institution almost perfectly in tune with the times. As a group dedicated to scientific medicine in the service of their community, they embodied the "three powerful themes of post-war life," identified by Rosemary Stevens in her book *In Sickness and In Wealth:* "the belief in the techniques of science as a liberating, rational solution to the problems of everyday existence; the importance of a sense of belonging, with growing emphasis on human relations; and 'togetherness,' fostered through membership in organized groups, activities and rituals."[23] Their prospects looked good.

Determined to open even though the building was still under construction, the partners toted an array of cleaning supplies into every corner of useable space and set about cleaning up the place. In the middle of the cleanup, a patient, attracted by the brand-new sign on the front of the building, came in with a minor complaint. Robert Green remembered being in mid-mop when he was approached by the medical center's first patient: "'Is there a doctor here?' the man wanted to know. I said, 'Yes, I'm a doctor.' He paused a bit while he reconciled what he was looking for with what he had found. It was some minor thing he needed to have wrapped up, so I wrapped him up and away he went."

FOUNDERS OF ST. LOUIS PARK MEDICAL CENTER
JULY 2, 1951

Arnold S. Anderson, Pediatrics
David M. Anderson, Urology
Alex Barno, Obstetrics/Gynecology
Donald W. Freeman, Obstetrics/Gynecology
Robert R. Geibink, Orthopedist
Sewell S. Gordon, Radiology
Robert A. (Bud) Green, Internal Medicine
Wyman E. Jacobson, Internal Medicine
John W. LaBree, Internal Medicine
George W. Lund, Pediatrics
Richard J. Webber, Surgery

7

THE PARTNERSHIP YEARS
ST. LOUIS PARK MEDICAL CENTER
1951 TO 1960

It is unlikely that there ever was or ever will be a better time to start a medical practice than the early 1950s. As basic science and research expanded understanding of human physiology, the physician, and more particularly the medical specialist, could offer hope and treatment where neither had been previously available. Open-heart surgery, for example, went from an interesting idea to accepted therapy. The tools required by medical specialists of the day were few and inexpensive, the demand for physicians was high, and the nation was entering a period of unprecedented growth in population and wealth.

For St. Louis Park Medical Center the timing may have been perfect, but success was far from assured. "They were a worried group in the beginning," Alvin L. Schultz, an internist who joined the group in 1954, recalled. "They were worried in part because they were not well accepted by the medical community, which thought their ideas were a form of communism, and in part because their whole financial futures were dependent on the clinic." According to Arnold Anderson, "The idea in those days was that if the child had a fever of over 101 or bled more than a teaspoon, you sent them to the Mayo Clinic or the university. That you could practice the ultimate in medicine in a suburban community was a totally foreign notion. We looked on ourselves as professionals who were searching for a better way to practice medicine."

This searching had created a unique clinic made up of skilled specialists who had sacrificed lucrative careers in private specialty practice to follow an ideal. With few independent physicians willing to refer their patients to a local multispecialty group, St. Louis Park Medical Center built its specialty practice from the ground up, offering primary care to a young, rapidly growing community. Patients soon began to come from the western half of Minneapolis, Hopkins, Edina, and St. Louis Park.

In the narrow corridors of St. Louis Park Medical Center, there was constant interaction and consultation on even routine cases. Schultz described the scene as follows: "The beauty of that small clinic building was [that it allowed us to do] a lot of curbstone diagnosis. I don't know how many times the OBs would say 'Do you want to feel a goiter?' and I would go down and feel the goiter and say 'This is a lump we'd better do something about' or 'This is one we won't worry about.' That interchange was really very good. It made me a better primary physician, and it made the obstetrician a better specialist."

Pediatrician George Lund recalled that this interaction was frequent, and unreimbursed. "I had a patient with a bleeding problem and I called Wyman [Jacobson] about it, late. He gave me advice over the phone, and when I got to work the next morning there were several pages of additional information on my desk. There was no gain for Wyman in that, but that's how it worked."[26]

This was group practice in a very real sense, and it carried over into the group's hospital practice as well. According to John LaBree, "Bud [Robert Green], Wyman, and I would make rounds together. Every morning we would go down to Mt. Sinai about eight o'clock, have a cup of coffee, and then make our rounds to see our patients. It was marvelous."

The group's close working relationship created opportunity to deemphasize, to some extent, the traditional doctor-patient relationship. The obstetricians, for instance, alternated calls so that patients would think of them as a group, instead of as individual, personal physicians. They also introduced handling deliveries on rotation. The internists, too, attempted to rotate their on-call duties. Not having to be constantly available to patients allowed the physicians to "have a livable life."[27]

As outgoing chief of staff, John LaBree wrote the following in 1954: "The clinic was born of a desire to serve our patients in the best possible manner, and to provide us with the means to enjoy our practice without sacrificing the character and quality of such care." This ideal was endangered he wrote by "our haste to build for the future, and in our constant effort to increase our economic yield. These dangers must not be allowed to harass us.... We must not lose sight of our ideals." Steps must be taken, he continued, to ensure growth "in a direction that carries with it a constant effort to maintain a high caliber of medical practice that gives every man a high sense of moral achievement and satisfaction. Let this always be firmly before us and let this clinic become great without becoming greedy."[28]

RESPONDING TO SUCCESS

Under the guidance of Wyman Jacobson, the group's first chief of staff, St. Louis Park Medical Center passed its first and most important test: It was still open after one year. Better than survival, however, was that by June 1952, the group doubled a partner's monthly draw, from $500 to $1,000 per month. By May 1953, the practice was growing steadily, with an average increase of nineteen new patients per day and an average increase in bookings of $1,000 per month over the month before.[29]

During the first few years, the group depended on "outside income" (up to 20 percent of their total revenues) from a variety of sources, including teaching positions at the university, a contract John LaBree had with the Dayton Company as its part-time medical director, and other speaking and consulting fees. As the patient base grew, this number shrank to less than 5 percent of total income by 1957.[30]

By mid-1952, several gaps in the group's practice had grown large enough to warrant addition of new physicians. Robert Koller became the group's first addition in December 1952 when he was chosen to head the new ear, nose, and throat (ENT) department. The ophthalmology department also got its start in late 1952 when R. E. Watson was brought in from the Veterans Administration Hospital

Dedicated to preserving the ideal of a co-equal partnership, St. Louis Park Medical Center conducted most business in regular meetings of the partnership. For the first several years each partner took a turn as chief of staff, but it soon became clear that some had more interest and aptitude in administration than others. By the end of the decade, consecutive terms became more the rule than the exception. To deal with the greater complexity of a rapidly growing clinic, which was always building or planning to build something, an executive committee was created in 1954 and consisted of the chief of staff and the department heads. Specific policy committees were also created on an as-needed basis.

on a part-time basis. In 1953, Titus P. Bellville, an obstetrician and clinical instructor at the university, began work at the clinic, taking over for Alex Barno who had been called for two years of active duty in the Army Medical Corps. One year later the group brought in a full-time ophthalmologist, Richard O. Leavenworth.

Pediatrics continued to grow rapidly. George Lund nominated Norman A. Sterrie, a decorated air squadron commander in World War II, for a position in the department in 1952. After struggling with his desire to practice in a smaller community, Sterrie joined the group in August 1953. However, even after Sterrie's arrival the pediatrics department was stretched to the limit. Consequently, the group recruited a fourth pediatrician, Roger I. Leinke, in September 1954, easing the caseload substantially. The relief was short-lived, however. In 1955, Leinke became the first new physician to decline a partnership, resigning to go into private practice. His departure put the department under tremendous pressure. In February 1956, George Lund reported to the board that none of the three pediatricians had been able to take their vacations during the past year, and none expected to have any time off until July 1956 when Richard T. Cushing was due to join the department. Cushing, a graduate of Yale Medical School, had been recruited by Arnold Anderson.

The one-man general-surgery department had also reached capacity. When Richard Webber recommended surgeon Frank E. Johnson, a classmate and former colleague at the Veterans Administration Hospital, as a potential new staff member, the group enthusiastically supported the choice. Johnson joined the group in October 1953 and quickly assumed a leadership role, succeeding David Anderson as chief of staff in 1956.

The growth of the clinic was not the only reason for change in the mid-1950s. The volume of radiological work generated by the clinic was far below what radiologist and founder Sewell Gordon felt he could handle. Well known in the community for his "roentgenological acumen," he had no trouble finding outside work.[31] Under the partnership agreement, this outside income was turned over to the group and divided equally. Gordon soon tired of this arrangement and somewhat reluctantly withdrew from the partnership in May 1954. The group missed his work, however, and eventually welcomed him back on a contract basis to head the radiological department, a position he held until 1974.

This time period also saw the arrival of Alvin Schultz, who was brought in to cover for Bud Green during an illness. TB-positive since childhood, Green was diagnosed with a tuberculoma in his left lung in 1954. Surgery to remove the lesion was to be followed by a six-month stay, in isolation, at the Veterans Administration Hospital. As he prepared for this extended absence, Green expressed heartfelt relief that "his practice would continue under the capable supervision of his partners."[32] "We had just bought a house on a contract, we had three kids and a fourth on the way. The clinic really saved the day for us, providing three months at full pay," Green recalled thirty years later.[33] Schultz, who at the time was on the faculty at the University of Minnesota Medical School, agreed to join the group temporarily. Not willing to abandon teaching entirely, Schultz continued as head of the Endocrine Clinic and returned to the university full-time in 1959.

Green returned to find the group in need of a fifth internist. He nominated his friend and fellow internist William Fifer, who in 1956 was finishing a Trudeau Teaching Fellowship at the university under Cecil Watson. "The appeal of the clinic was I could stay on the faculty at the university and keep teaching one-half day a week," Fifer explained, adding that though he had intended to remain in academic medicine he never regretted his decision.

The group's first business manager, John Fields, left in mid-1953 and was replaced by Richard E. Anderson. A former Air Force flight instructor and a former manager for Arid-Air,

Anderson brought an added measure of business experience to the department.[34]

TO GROW OR NOT

As the new medical center raced to keep up with the demand for medical services in fast-growing St. Louis Park, a quiet struggle developed over the group's direction. Some in the group were wholeheartedly committed to enlarging the clinic to its potential. Richard Webber told the group in 1953 that their goals should "always be pushed back, for it is in the creative portion of life that satisfaction lies." Failure to meet the challenge presented by the burgeoning demand for services would "mean the clinic has failed in its civic mission."[35]

Others were not so sure. Partners with strong ties to teaching and other outside activities were beginning to feel the pressure to keep longer hours at the clinic because their patients were impatient with anything less than full-time access to their own physicians. As the staff grew to seventeen in 1955, many of the physicians began to feel nostalgia for the smaller group. Saturday luncheons at Culbertson's Restaurant, an informal tradition established early on, were becoming unwieldy. For Alvin Schultz the lunches were "part social and part business. We ironed out our differences. It was a beautiful . . . relationship, which couldn't last." According to Arnold Anderson, "We spent a lot of hours debating growth, because the thing was growing and we didn't want to grow."

Other growth-related issues were discussed at length throughout the mid-1950s. From what area should the medical center accept patients? Should the group continue to add pediatricians and internists in response to community needs or place more emphasis on the specialty and subspecialty work for which the staff had trained—the work that might "utilize to best advantage the unique talents of this group"?[36]

Ultimately, Webber's concept of "civic mission" held sway. The group would, as the minutes of February 1956 record, "accept growth wherever it occurred naturally and without particular reference to the income of a particular specialty. If the community needed pediatricians, then pediatricians would be added."[37]

Acceptance of growth, however, was not enough to bring in the referrals necessary to keep the subspecialists busy. After serving for a year as chief of staff, Frank Johnson resigned in the fall of 1956, citing growing pessimism of ever developing an active practice in thoracic surgery within the clinic. "I have," he told the group, "weighed my desire to practice the specialty for which I have trained, on the one hand, against the joy, pleasure, and financial security of practicing with this excellent and congenial group."[38] He went on to found the Minnesota Thoracic Group, a successful private surgical practice in Minneapolis, and was instrumental in creating the Children's Heart Fund, a program to bring children from the Third World to the United States for heart surgery. Forty years after his resignation from St. Louis Park Medical Center, Johnson remembered it was the resistance of his friends in the medical community that forced a decision. "Friends outside found it impossible to refer to me, because they were afraid they would lose not just their patient [to the clinic], but their patient's family as well."

A conversation between Arnold Anderson, who became chief of staff in 1958, and Harry Harwick of the Mayo Foundation helped the group face some of the more unpleasant aspects of continuous growth. Presented with the young group's dilemma, Harwick told Anderson, "You think the Mayos ever wanted to grow? We finally decided that it was worse not to grow than to grow, because if you put the brakes on the organization, you create an attitude of negativism throughout the whole organization. . . . So if you are in a growth phase it's inevitable, and you had better just go with it, if you want to practice the medicine you want to practice."[39]

BRICKS AND MORTAR

However the group felt about growth, by the mid-1950s it had overtaken them. The space they had designed in 1950 to accommodate the minimum needs of the eleven founders was by 1955 housing seventeen physicians. As early as April 1953, the partnership was considering expansion seriously enough to declare all "unnecessary expenses tabled for the next twelve months," in hopes of building a capital reserve fund.[40]

By 1955 the overcrowding could no longer be tolerated. Business Manager Richard Anderson told the group that the phenomenal growth over the past year had created a situation where "schedules were badly overcrowded for days at a time . . . [with] the girls at the appointment desk . . . spending more time trying to keep people away from the clinic than in trying to give service to people."[41]

A building committee, headed by Norman Sterrie, presented a plan to add 6,000 square feet under the existing space. Pediatrics, ENT, and the eye department would move to the basement to allow the other departments to expand on the first floor. The group approved the plan in late 1955. Further study identified the need to reorient the entrance to the south and expand business-office space. A two-story addition extending to the south of the waiting area was the solution.

Construction in 1957 was preceded by the laborious hand digging of the basement, aided by a system of conveyors. Not excavating a full basement under the medical center, a cost-saving move in 1950, became the costly mistake Morten Arneson had predicted. The Prudential Life

Insurance Company financed the addition's cost of $144,000, about $20,000 more than the cost of the original building. Another $51,000 was provided for equipment and for the purchase of the land under the existing building,[42] for which Arneson had given the group a ten-year option to buy at $20,000. When the group exercised the option in 1956, the value of that 100 feet of land on Excelsior Boulevard had risen to well over $50,000, another example of the many contributions the Arnesons made to ensure the clinic's success.[43]

NEW SPACE, NEW ENERGY

The move into the new "ground floor" in July 1957 provided a welcome relief from the bottlenecks and overcrowding. Recruiting again picked up. Pediatrics, which had moved into the new space with four physicians, soon added a fifth, Donnell D. Etzwiler, another Yale graduate. Obstetrics moved into the space vacated by pediatrics and, in 1959, added Melvin P. Baken Jr., a graduate of the University of Minnesota in both dentistry and obstetrics. (Baken joined the group after working for a year with his father at the Nicollet Clinic.) Internal medicine moved into the former obstetrics suite and added two new physicians: Jack A. Vennes in 1957 and David A. Randall in 1959. Surgery remained in its original location on the first floor and added Jerome T. Grismer and Robert B. Benjamin in 1957.

The new physicians brought with them new energy—energy the group sought to use to its fullest potential. Each new member was formally invited to participate at all levels in the organization, with the hope that the new physicians would accept the ideals and spirit of the group as their own. "The group had a very generous attitude towards the young people coming in," Norman Sterrie noted, an attitude he felt was key to the clinic's rapid growth.

A HOSPITAL IN ST. LOUIS PARK

The growth of St. Louis Park Medical Center during the 1950s matched the growth of the surrounding community. St. Louis Park, a boomtown of young World War II veterans and their families, was well on the way to doubling its population during the medical center's first ten years. Although it was not a wealthy community, the average family income in the "Park" was significantly higher than the average for the city of Minneapolis or statewide.[44] Since the late 1940s, residents of the growing suburb had been trying to organize a hospital for their community. This effort was abandoned in 1954, when Asbury Methodist Hospital, then located in downtown Minneapolis, chose a site on Excelsior Boulevard, less than a mile west of St. Louis Park Medical Center, for its new location.

The medical center was excited about the prospect of a new hospital in the western suburbs. Robert Green, in a letter to the *St. Louis Park Dispatch*, urged "Parkers" to support Asbury's plans to locate in St. Louis Park: "The advantages of proximity for prompt, efficient hospital care for suburban dwellers, and for the thousands who work here, are obvious."[45] Construction on the new hospital, which was to be called "Methodist Hospital," began in the spring of 1957.

When Methodist opened its doors on February 16, 1959, the convenience of the five-minute commute to the new state-of-the-art facility overwhelmed the history of mutual support and cooperation the physicians had experienced with Mt. Sinai Hospital. All but a few of the physicians soon transferred their hospital practice to Methodist. The physician staff at the new hospital elected Robert Green president of the medical staff in 1960, and at least thirteen other St. Louis Park Medical Center physicians served as department chairs or committee members that year.

MANAGING CHANGE

As early as 1954, it was becoming clear that the original partnership structure could not support the growth overtaking the group. The management systems adequate in 1952, when the clinic's total income was $217,000, were strained to the breaking point in 1957, when revenues topped $701,000.[46]

When Arnold Anderson accepted his election to head the group in December 1957, his words set the tone for his tenure: "I won't pretend I'm not surprised and honored to have been chosen for a turn at this responsibility at this time. I was thrilled to become a member of the clinic in the first place, and tonight, though my flesh is tired and my frame is sagging, the thrill of working with you men is still fresh and strong in me. . . . I never forget for a moment that many of the opportunities for community service and personal development I have enjoyed come to me as a direct result of this association. . . . At this juncture, it seems to me, we need to redefine our larger purpose in the practice of medicine; we need to grasp a new vision of our role in the whole medical community, and it may be that we shall have to discover and develop new techniques for arriving at our mutual aims."[47]

Looking to the future, Anderson urged the group to "take time now to appraise and rechart our course. We have all known plenty of enterprises that run out of steam before the second generation. We need now, forgive me, to anticipate and plan to thwart the symptoms of our own middle age. . . . This started as a cooperative venture," he stated, "and will always do best as a cooperative venture. . . . Together, we should be able to evolve a program worthy of 1958."

Anderson laid out several areas that might yield new opportunities for growth and development and community service: "What we *must* do is discover a way to exploit each man's capabilities to the utmost, in the interests of the man himself, the clinic, and the community they both serve."[48] Anderson then concluded, with notable understatement, "Certainly, in the area of income and expense we are faced with a challenge."[49]

It was this challenge of "income and expense" that became top priority. Growing dissatisfaction with partnership income and a construction-related shortfall in early 1958 forced the group to begin investigating each area of the practice, looking for and implementing cost-saving measures ranging from reducing physician salaries by one-third to turning out the lights in empty offices. The Personnel Committee, led by William Fifer, implemented a "work-smarter-not-harder" program, which attempted to increase production in each department by giving employees supervisory status and the responsibility to create production standards.

By May 1958, Arnold Anderson had become frustrated with inexperience in the business office and a business structure that "helped make it impossible for Richard Anderson to discharge adequately the responsibility of management."[50] The Executive Committee recommended that the position of business manager be eliminated and a new position of executive secretary to the Executive Committee be created. This position was offered to Richard Anderson for a trial period of ninety days, but the problems undermining the business office remained, and Richard Anderson resigned in September 1958.

Faced with hiring a new executive, Arnold Anderson asked his business mentor David Babcock of Dayton's personnel department to help screen the applicants for relevant business and executive experience. Of the twenty-one applicants, one stood out. J. Roger Asplin, an executive with Freuhoff Trucking in South Bend, Indiana, and an administrator with a military hospital during World War II, had the solid business experience the group was looking for. He began work at the medical center in December 1958 realizing only then that the executive secretary, in practice, was in a very weak position. Asplin recounted, "They had had what they thought was a poor experience in medical administration, [so] they had appointed doctors in charge of personnel, the business office, accounting, and supplies. I had to reintroduce them to the concept of a responsible administrator. Arnie [Anderson] understood this pretty well, so eventually the doctors drifted away to the point where I could absorb all the management functions and did."

REORGANIZATION

Asplin arrived at an important time. After more than five years of discussion and study, St. Louis Park Medical Center was about to make the first major change in its organizational structure.

Since 1952, the group had been discussing ways to separate the ownership in the buildings from the ownership of the medical practice. Intent on creating a democratically controlled association of physicians, the group realized that the accumulation and appreciation of physical assets would make it increasingly difficult to recruit young, research-oriented physicians, who would expect, but could not afford, to purchase an equal share in the partnership. In 1954, Richard Anderson and William Green, the group's attorney and Bud Green's brother, had urged the partnership to reorganize as a Massachusetts trust. This would create an unincorporated association controlled by a managing board for the benefit of its members, which offered the advantages of a corporation, but avoided the state prohibition on the incorporation of physician groups. However, in 1954, keeping up with the increased patient load and expanding the original building took precedence over more long-term management issues.

In early 1958, at essentially the same time the Nicollet Clinic was making the decision to reorganize as a professional association, the various shortcomings in the business affairs of the medical center became painfully obvious. Sensing the need for a thorough report, Arnold Anderson appointed Wyman Jacobson to head a committee to examine the organization and "formulate a plan for a table of organization, to define the responsibilities of the Executive Committee and other areas of responsibility." In Anderson's words, "From a governance standpoint we were at a log jam."

By October 1958, the committee was ready with a proposal for reorganization of the partnership. Jacobson's report outlined the tax and management advantages of reorganization and proposed several alternatives. After "considerable discussion," the partnership unanimously approved the committee's plan to prepare articles of incorporation for a new building corporation and articles of association for an operational trust.[51]

At regular meetings over the next year with Roger Asplin and William Green, the committee hammered out the details. The buildings and land would transfer to the building corporation, Medcenter, Inc. Stock in the corporation would transfer to the partners in amounts equal to their share of the book value of the real estate, with a cap on ownership equal to the largest single holding. The cash and equipment would transfer to the operational trust, the St. Louis Park Medical Center, a business trust. Certificates in the trust were split into two classes, voting and nonvoting. Each partner would receive two voting shares, and twenty-eight nonvoting shares. To maintain an equal ownership in the trust, each new member would be required to purchase twenty-eight nonvoting shares, and all shares would be surrendered on leaving the association. Each partner would become an employee of the medical center.

Perhaps most important for the future, the reorganization plan centralized management functions of the medical center in a five-member board elected by the beneficiaries of the business trust and allowed leadership to be reelected to the board without restriction, encouraging a new continuity and development of leadership. The agreement and declaration of trust was approved on December 31, 1959, officially establishing a new era at St. Louis Park Medical Center. Wyman Jacobson was selected by the group to be the first president of the trust. The partnership that had created a working institution from the ideals and goals of eleven young physicians was quietly dissolved in favor of an organization that might more ably carry those ideals forward.

OF IDEALS AND OBJECTIVES

Although the group's ideals were "mutually accepted and fanatically adhered to," they hadn't been properly set down prior to 1957.[52] In the months before taking over from his friend Robert Green as chief of staff, Arnold Anderson set a condition on his acceptance. He would take the position if Green would write and present a formal statement of the group's ideals and objectives. Green accepted the challenge. His "Statement of Objectives," formally adopted by the group in November 1957, read as follows:

> The Saint Louis Park Medical Center was organized in the belief that group practice offers the best opportunity to promote and maintain the highest standards of medical proficiency.
>
> It is our aim that each member preserve his own identity but at the same time share his resources and experience with the others in the group for their mutual benefit and the benefit of all who come here for medical care.
>
> It is our hope that we may reflect credit on our community in which we work and live, and by maintaining high standards in our practice of medicine contribute to the health and enrich the lives of those around us.
>
> Finally and not least of our goals is the desire to contribute, individually and together, to the advancement of medical science through research and education.[53]

These words were committed to bronze and hung in the waiting area of the medical center. They carried the group through their first major reorganization and served thereafter as a yardstick and a guide as the medical center grew and changed.

8

EXCEEDING EXPECTATIONS

ST. LOUIS PARK MEDICAL CENTER

1961 TO 1970

THE 1960S DAWNED FULL OF PROMISE. THE EXPLOSIVE postwar growth in the U.S. economy had created high expectations for the future. The dark cloud of the Cold War and the initial terror of atomic weapons had been molded into the more manageable, rationalized framework of "mutually assured destruction." Polio, tuberculosis, and a multitude of bacterial infections had been largely controlled. Medical science was creating new diagnostic machines and new treatment technologies daily. Kidney dialysis, for example, provided the difference between life and death for a small but growing number of patients in the early 1960s. The autoanalyzer, invented in 1957, was bringing unheard of accuracy to laboratory blood testing. The secrets of human chromosomes were slowly revealing themselves to researchers. Computerized information systems were offering a glimpse of what might be possible in clinical recordkeeping.

St. Louis Park Medical Center had much to celebrate on its tenth anniversary in 1961. The staff had grown steadily to include twenty-six specialists. Referrals accounted for 6 to 7 percent of the total patient count, evidence of the group's growing stature among their peers.[54] The primary care specialists—internists, obstetricians, and pediatri-

"Make no little plans, they have no magic to stir men's blood."

Unknown (favorite quote of Wyman E. Jacobson, M.D.)

cians—were extremely busy and patient loyalty was high. Future growth seemed assured as the group's loyal patient base in the west metro area grew and grew older.

ELLERBE EXPANSION PROGRAM

There are few more obvious measures of the growth of an organization than its building program. St. Louis Park Medical Center in the 1960s was no exception. The steady growth in staff size and patient visits quickly overwhelmed the basement expansion of 1956. The quiet, easy-going atmosphere of the early 1950s gave way to a bustling, sometimes jostling, group practice perennially short of parking space, examining rooms, and office space. More land and more office space were essential.

Focused as they were on recruiting, teaching, and practicing medicine, the group had never articulated a vision of the physical plant required to meet the expansive goals of their mission statement. Arnold Anderson, in his second year as chief of staff, convinced the group to hire Robby Kerr, a well-known physician and architect with Ellerbe Architects, to analyze the group's growth and future space needs. In September 1959, Kerr presented a draft long-range building plan, the first essential of which was securing a site large enough to include the required buildings, parking, and open space. Subsequently, two options for securing the needed land were explored: purchasing the adjoining Arneson property to the east or purchasing a vacant site across Excelsior Boulevard from Methodist Hospital. Reluctant to finance an entirely new clinic, the group decided to approach the Arnesons.

A few years after the medical center had been built, Morten and Katheren Arneson had closed their nursery and built a grocery store on the corner of Excelsior Boulevard and Quentin Avenue. In 1959, the Arnesons were leasing the building to the National Tea Company.

However, thinking about retiring from some of their business enterprises, the Arnesons were ready to sell the land and building to the group.

The terms the Arnesons accepted on January 1, 1960, were yet another example of their generosity toward the medical center. Medcenter, Inc., the clinic's property company, would make no down payment and, over the next fifteen years, pay only an annual stipend of $18,000 to the Arnesons. The annual payment was roughly three-quarters of the property's lease value. Any balance remaining upon the Arnesons' deaths would be paid to the St. Louis Park Medical Center Research Foundation. The purchase of this property for long-term growth, however, did nothing to relieve the existing crowded conditions in the clinic, since National Tea's lease allowed the company to remain in the building for another three years.

With the site chosen, Ellerbe prepared an expansion plan that included a six-story building attached to the west side of the existing clinic on Excelsior Boulevard and a smaller, 5,000-square-foot addition to the north of the clinic to be built immediately to handle current overcrowding. The plan for the multistory clinic required the acquisition of a lot immediately west of the existing building, and a long-term lease was arranged in the fall of 1961.

North and South Expansion

While the details of the long-range building plan were being worked out, the pressure for additional space was increasing rapidly. Internal medicine, the largest department, had grown to eight physicians. New-patient registrations had begun to drop as serious appointment delays turned patients away. In May 1961, the board gave Ellerbe the go-ahead to add 35 feet to the north, the first phase of the expansion plan. Construction began on October 24 and was completed in the spring of 1962. The new space included sixteen rooms on the first floor for the internal medicine and obstetrics/gynecology departments and ten rooms on the ground floor for the ear, nose, and throat and eye departments.

The building project at this time included creating additional underground space in front of the waiting area (at the north end of the building) for the new Arneson Library and record rooms. An entry walk/patio was laid over this area.

Obstetrics and Gynecology Addition

By the spring of 1964, growth had again raced ahead of the planning process. Numerous problems had emerged to stall plans for development on the Arneson nursery site. Finding enough room for parking and overcoming the objections of homeowners on the block were two of the most perplexing. Dissatisfied with Ellerbe's approach to the project, the group hired a new firm to design a suite for the obstetrics/gynecology department.[55] Built over the library and designed by Setter, Leach & Lindstrom, Inc., the suite included six examining rooms, four offices, a waiting room, and a nurses station. Construction of the obstetrics addition was partially financed by patients through the direct purchase of corporate bonds. The business department, borrowing a successful strategy from Bachman's Florists, inserted flyers in patients' bills, informing them of the opportunity to purchase the bonds.[56]

During this same time period, the architects continued to develop plans for a multistory addition on the original nursery site. In November 1965, the board approved a five-story plan of some 45,000 square feet.

Pediatric Annex

The grocery-store building became available for expansion in late 1963, when National Tea vacated the building. Much to Morten Arneson's dismay, the group decided that turning the grocery store into clinical space was an inadequate, short-term solution to a long-term problem. Early in 1964, the store was leased to a new grocer, Hove's. Several years later Arneson admitted to Alex Barno, "I had never had anything hurt me so bad,"[57] and it wouldn't be the last time Arneson and "his group" had differences over business strategies. The clinic's relationship with Arneson was salvaged in 1965, however, when Hove's went out of business. This time, with plans for a new clinic building still stalled, the board asked Setter, Leach & Lindstrom, Inc. to remodel the grocery building into a state-of-the-art pediatrics department.

In all, 6,600 square feet, three times its previous space, were renovated for the pediatrics department, and an additional 5,400 square feet were converted for use by the allergy clinic and the new data processing department. A heated connection between the two buildings was also completed at this time.

CROSSING THE BOULEVARD

For nearly six years the group's plans for a new major medical office complex were stymied by their inability to acquire enough land around the original nursery site to accommodate the traffic such a building would generate. City plans to convert the Excelsior Boulevard corridor into "downtown" St. Louis Park, including municipal parking to serve the proposed larger clinic, kept the group focused on the former nursery site for several years. But after several tries, the city redevelopment plans collapsed.

In June 1966, with no assistance from the city on the horizon, the medical center board authorized Medcenter, Inc., to purchase the site of the former Beltline Pay Dump, one block straight north of the clinic on 39th Street. Although it lacked direct access to Excelsior Boulevard or

Route 100 and appeared "out of the way," the six-acre property had the distinct advantage of having ample room for patient parking and future growth.[58] Once this property was acquired, the idea of squeezing a large medical building onto the original three-acre site was quickly abandoned. The board, with Wyman Jacobson serving as president and chairman, voted unanimously in September 1966 to move across Excelsior Boulevard.

The plans Setter, Leach & Lindstrom, Inc. had developed in 1964 for the nursery site were now resurrected, with modifications, for a building on the new site. The five-story structure would have a dramatic, exposed concrete framework, outlining tall, narrow windows and red-brick wall panels. The foundation, which included a basement and subbasement, was built solidly enough to support twelve stories, an expression in concrete of the group's hopes for the future. Early in the planning process, Wyman Jacobson dubbed the new building the "Northland Building," and the name stuck.

Preconstruction planning continued through most of 1967 under the guidance of Norman Sterrie and Richard Webber. The long, cooperative planning process yielded many innovations that benefitted the group. For example, the tall, narrow windows in each examining room preserved both the natural light and the patient's privacy. The two lower floors had ten-foot-high ceilings to accommodate the newest X-ray equipment. A system called the Tele-lift—automated carts traveling by rail in hidden tunnels—connected the record room in the basement with nurses stations on each floor. A new phone system allowed each phone to have its own extension number.

Farmers and Mechanics Bank approved $2.5 million in construction financing in August 1967. Knutson Construction Co., Inc. was selected as the general contractor and construction began immediately. By this time the group was in a big hurry to complete the project. Construction of the shell started in September 1967, before the interior finish drawings were complete. Close supervision and "on-the-job decision making" saved six to nine months, by Roger Asplin's estimate. "At times it was hard for the architect to keep ahead of the builder."[59]

On October 20, 1968, the original clinic building on Excelsior Boulevard was dedicated to Morten and Katheren Arneson. The couple, who had done so much to support the group, were presented with a set of golden keys by Richard Webber. "You held the keys to our future," he said during the ceremony, "and you hold the keys to our heart." Since the new building would not have enough finished space for the entire practice, the group planned to retain the "Arneson Building" for the allergy, ophthalmology, obstetrics, and other departments as needed.

Knutson Construction proved to be very efficient and cost conscious, which allowed a sixth story to be shelled in. In all, 102 medical office and examining rooms were completed, tripling the office space available to the 51 physicians and 200 employees working at the medical center.[60] Departments moved into their new accommodations as space was finished and, with the aid of Wyman Jacobson's "equipment bible," which identified the placement of every piece of furniture and equipment, the move was completed on December 15, 1968. In January, St. Louis Park Medical Center welcomed more than 2,500 guests at four open-house events.[61]

Norman Sterrie introduced into the Northland plans many features to aid handicapped patients. "This was the era before handicap-access laws," Sterrie recalled, "so this sort of thing got done only if someone took an interest. I happened to have a handicapped person, a lawyer, in my practice, and he agreed to spend some time with me going over the plans to make the new building more accessible. I came back with a long list for the architects. Even so, after we were in Northland for a while we discovered that a frail person or someone with a broken arm could not open the front doors and we had to replace them. Aside from that, I thought we did a pretty good job."

MANAGING GROWTH

For the clinic's leaders during the 1960s, growth was not simply possible, it was absolutely necessary. "Since a professional service also has a natural life cycle," Wyman Jacobson told the group in 1966, "it is inexcusable to not protect its progress. It is necessary to ward off every evidence of decline and start new upward movements as the

"The continuous addition of highly skilled staff keeps us on our toes and keeps us moving restlessly ahead. As long as we have the continuing stimulus of association with these new men, continue to develop our own and group professional programs and continue to fulfill our commitments to the University teaching and training programs, we will grow professionally and maintain the position of excellence we have achieved to date."
Robert Green, M.D., Annual Report of the Medical Staff Committee, *1970*

only certain protection for future profits and professional growth."[62]

By all accounts, recruiting was the key to promoting "new upward movements." From 1966 to 1971 the group grew by twenty-six full-time physicians. Although there was a general shortage of physicians at the time, St. Louis Park Medical Center was able to fill specialty slots once a need was determined. Its growing national reputation for research and academic work attracted high-level talent.

One result of attracting talent was the difficulty of maintaining a uniform top-pay schedule. As early as 1963, the board had recognized "individual differences in age, skill, energy, health, family responsibilities, and earning capacity." The challenge was to recognize differences in productivity without compromising the commitment to professional education and academic time. The variable-pay schedule, implemented in 1963 and revised in 1966, provided the answer.

Earl Young, a surgeon who had joined the clinic in 1960, became chair of the Professional Compensation Committee. Under his judicious eye, four funds were established out of which each individual's total compensation was drawn. The largest fund, accounting for 45 percent of the total available for salaries, was allocated in proportion to the base salary. The second fund, 20 percent of the total, was allocated based on the individual's bookings, recognizing extra effort and the high-and-growing earning potential of some of the specialties. The third fund, also 20 percent, was allocated based on individual achievement as determined by the committee's review of the physician's activity report. This process allowed academic achievement, publications, and research work to be recognized. Finally, a smaller amount was allocated to provide the "flexibility to recognize any and all special situations."[63]

Looking back, Wyman Jacobson said this "very unusual" compensation system "attracted good physicians and provided a base for the growth which has been so phenomenal." The system was summed up another way in a wisecrack Alex Barno attributed to Jacobson: "Your bonus increase becomes effective the moment you do."[64]

ADMINISTRATIVE MATURITY

Managing the growth curve during this period became the primary preoccupation of the administrative committees and Administrator Roger Asplin. Unable to raise the capital needed to expand facilities or finance academic programs through the stock market as a public corporation might do, the board knew that any growth would have to be planned carefully—both to maintain physician income and to address the financial concerns of the growing list of creditors resulting from building construction.

Arnold Anderson and Asplin introduced comprehensive budgeting in the early 1960s to ensure that costs and fee schedules were examined and that long-term needs were projected for each department. Addressing the group in 1962, Anderson observed that the development of a comprehensive budget "is hard, painful, and time consuming. . . . We must now maintain and improve these systems if we are to maintain professional excellence."[65] According to Asplin, "We asked each of the department heads to estimate what they thought their production was going to be and administration took care of the rest. . . . We were amazingly on target."

The administrative capability of the group grew by leaps and bounds under Asplin, Anderson, and Jacobson, with sophisticated budgeting being just one example. But Anderson's goal of establishing a clinic-wide, standard fee schedule remained illusive. It wasn't until the early 1970s that the staff physicians finally let go of their traditional prerogative to set the fees they charged for each procedure. Computerization of records and finances in the late 1960s, which allowed the group to track service much more closely, made the argument for a standard fee schedule—administered by the business office—persuasive. The management challenge, Asplin told the board in 1969, was to meet "the problems of growth and costs on the one hand and the pressures from government and society for the delivery of more comprehensive medical care at a reasonable cost."[66]

COMPUTERIZATION

A minirevolution occurred in management technology during the mid-1960s, and St. Louis Park Medical Center rushed to the front lines. As early as 1962, the administration was planning to convert to computerized accounting. In April 1964, Roger Asplin helped organize a data processing institute at the Mayo Clinic for the National Association of Clinic Managers. This experience, Asplin told the group, "awakened me to the fact [that computerization] would possibly be the most earth-shaking of any [administrative change] we have made."[67]

In 1965 the new data processing department installed a used IBM punch-card machine for processing bills. It cut the time needed to process statements by three to five days. The punch-card system, outdated almost before it was installed, was soon replaced by a Univac 9200, the group's first in-house computer. When program-driven software became available in 1969, diagnosis coding of statements was one of the first programs installed—"a dream come true" for the Records Committee. For the first time, information on diagnoses and procedures was in permanent computer storage and available for clinical research programs. By 1970 the data processing department was processing 20,000 patient statements per month.[68]

EXPANDING THE PRACTICE

Throughout the 1960s, St. Louis Park Medical Center added new departments, which broadened the traditional definition of the multispecialty clinic. Some of the new departments resulted from the addition of a physician trained in a new specialty. The dermatology department, for instance, was created in 1966 when Edwin Rice joined the group. Other departments, such as the allergy department, were created to give independent status to a group of subspecialists already working in another department. The new departments enlarged the clinic's reputation as a one-stop medical center.

Department of Industrial Medicine

Between 1951 and 1965, individual physicians within the group contracted with local industries—including Dayton's, Supervalu Stores, and the Tennant Company—to provide annual executive and preemployment physicals. Hoping to establish a more direct line of communication with local industry, the group hired Herschel Perlman, a general practitioner and president of the Methodist Hospital medical staff, to create a department of industrial medicine in 1968. The industrial medicine department consolidated routine physician services to area businesses and government into one department.

The Department of Industrial Medicine became the Department of Occupational Medicine in 1975 to better reflect the range of services offered. In addition to routine physicals, these services included assistance with workplace safety, environmental health, emergency care, and medical planning.

Family Practice Department

In April 1969, William Fifer, chief recruiter for the medical center, asked Harley Racer, an experienced general practitioner, to set up a department of family practice that would "specialize" in giving primary care to the clinic's adult patients. Prior to this, internists—especially ones new to the group—were generally assigned the task of treating sore throats, backaches, and other routine illnesses. The new family medicine department got an immediate boost from the patients who followed Racer from his Bloomington practice. A second physician, Ronald Ohmann, was added in May 1969. By the end of 1969, the department had seen 3 percent of the clinic's patients, a number that would rise steadily through the 1970s to reach 13 percent in 1977.[69]

Years of discussion and controversy preceded the establishment of the family practice department. A large number of the medical center's physicians considered family medicine to be inferior to their academically oriented subspecialties. A multispecialty clinic, by definition, did not include general or family practitioners, the argument went. At the same time, the medical center was facing increasing pressure from patients who wanted to be able to get all their care at the clinic. There was also a growing national movement to recognize family medicine as a specialty in itself and to establish a national certification program. These developments, combined with internists' complaints about having to treat a steady stream of unspectacular cases, had convinced Fifer to turn to Racer to create a model for family practice.

In addition to setting up a department of family practice within the multispecialty clinic, Harley Racer was asked to plan and implement a residency program affiliated with the University of Minnesota. Dr. Racer welcomed his first "trainee physician," Margit Winstrom, in August 1969. Winstrom became the first woman physician to hold a full-time position on the staff at St. Louis Park Medical Center. The family practice residency was the second university-affiliated residency program—the first being the surgical residency program—housed at the medical center, a notable achievement for a private group clinic.

Family Counseling and Social Services Department

Pressure to provide a comprehensive range of primary care services also drove the creation of the Department of Social Services and Family Counseling in 1969. The pediatrics department provided developmental support to the new department, and Budrowe Larson, a social worker, was hired to organize and head the effort. The department grew quickly to include three full-time counselors by 1970.

The position of "patient counselor" was created in 1968. Cassel Wherland, a registered nurse with many years of service at the medical center, was stationed at a desk near the main waiting area. She helped patients find their way quickly to the right physician or health service, answered phone inquiries from worried patients, helped to arrange appointments with the appropriate specialists, and registered emergency cases. The new "patient services" was unique enough in the medical profession to warrant notice by the Minneapolis Tribune *in 1971. Patients often called Wherland directly because they appreciated her willingness to "hear their story out. She gives them a feeling of security and a sense that there is someone out there who cares about their problems."*[70]

CLINICAL INNOVATIONS

The group's commitment to research and training created a dynamic atmosphere where innovative programs were proposed and allowed to go forward with only one condition—that the program be studied in detail as to its effectiveness for the patient and its impact on the clinic's finances. Very often these new programs were developed by newly recruited members of the group who, with fresh energy and smaller practices, seized the opportunity to serve the greater interest of the group and the group's patients. This liberal attitude toward the independent contribution of the younger physicians, an important factor in the group's ability to attract high-quality talent, added to the whirlwind of important innovations to and expansions of the medical center's clinical services throughout the 1960s.

Pediatric and Adult Cardiology Clinics

As the practice and the reputations of the individual specialists grew, new consultation clinics were created. George Lund developed a statewide pediatric cardiology practice, holding weekly clinics for the state Crippled Children's Service, examining children with heart murmurs, and doing referrals as needed. At that time only three places in

Minnesota were doing pediatric cardiology: the Mayo Clinic, the University of Minnesota, and St. Louis Park Medical Center. Lund obtained his subspecialty certification in pediatric cardiology in 1963, a title generally reserved for physicians in academic institutions.

The adult cardiologists, John LaBree and James C. Dahl, and thoracic surgeon Jerome T. Grismer established a federally funded regional heart catheterization laboratory at Mt. Sinai Hospital in 1964. Four years later the St. Louis Park Medical Center cardiology department organized a similar facility at Methodist Hospital. The apparent "extravagance" of this duplication was dictated, Dahl reported to the board in 1969, by the "unstable nature of Mt. Sinai politics" and the need to create a large referral base to support a growing cardiovascular surgery program.[71]

The thoracic surgery program grew steadily under Grismer, following his return from advanced training in July 1963. Using the facilities at Mt. Sinai, Grismer completed seven open-heart surgery cases in 1963 and fourteen in 1964, accounting for the bulk of the cardiac cases seen by the Mt. Sinai staff as well as of his own group. A second thoracic surgeon, David E. Raab, joined the group in 1965, boosting the number of open-heart surgeries to thirty-seven for the year.

Telemetric EKG

As a referral clinic for many general practice physicians in greater Minnesota, St. Louis Park Medical Center was alert to the new opportunities afforded by the emerging communications technologies. The first was a unique cardiology clinic proposed and organized by cardiologist James Dahl, a partner since 1959. Using a new telephone interface introduced by Medtronic, Inc., Dahl set up a system to transmit electrocardiogram (EKG) readings from remote locations. Physicians in a community hospital could administer an EKG that, in turn, could be interpreted immediately by the cardiology specialists hundreds of miles away at the medical center.

After receiving approval from the board, Dahl installed the first sending unit at Hutchinson Community Hospitals, in Hutchinson, Minnesota, in January 1962. The service grew slowly during the next few years, but by 1969 medical center cardiologists were reading over three thousand tracings each year from six hospitals in two states. Improvements in the system, including a portable receiving unit, allowed the cardiology department to interpret over six thousand remote EKGs in 1970 from thirty-eight hospitals. This was the bookings equivalent of one full-time cardiologist.

Coronary care in the mid-1960s was no job for a physician who liked regular hours. John LaBree recalls that while the early coronary care units dramatically increased the survival of heart patients, they also added tremendously to the workload of the cardiologist. When the units were new, nurses and residents weren't experienced with the equipment, so "any blip on the cardiogram would trigger a call to me, and we would have to run out there in the middle of the night. There were three of us and we were getting killed." Jerome Grismer noted with some understatement in 1965 the "rugged schedule" observed by the cardiac surgeons, who at that time routinely stayed at the hospital for forty-eight hours after an open-heart surgery.[72]

Kidney Dialysis at Methodist Hospital

Patients suffering from acute kidney failure at Methodist Hospital got a second chance at life in 1962, thanks in part to another young physician, Donald A. Duncan, pursuing his academic interests at the medical center. Duncan had worked on the University of Minnesota's Artificial Kidney Team as a resident. He became the director of the Methodist Hospital program upon joining St. Louis Park Medical Center in 1962. Methodist Hospital's dialysis unit was a first for the private hospitals in the region. After several dramatic successes with trauma patients, the unit began to work with patients who had lost kidney function and were facing long-term dialysis. By 1972, Duncan and his new medical center colleague, Henry Smith, were seeing 275 dialysis patients per month at the Methodist Artificial Kidney Center.

Diabetes Education Center

When Donnell Etzwiler joined the pediatrics department in 1957, he chose as his academic project the study of pediatric diabetes at the University of Minnesota Endocrine Clinic. At the clinic he worked with a series of young diabetics who were repeatedly returning to the hospital with complications brought on by their diabetes. From these encounters, Etzwiler concluded that lack of good information, not lack of science, was holding back the effective treatment of diabetes, exacting a tremendous cost on patients in terms of complications and shortened lives, and costing the community millions of dollars in unnecessary hospitalization.

In October 1965, Etzwiler asked the medical center board to allow him to spend up to 50 percent of his time developing a new regional diabetes education center to train physicians, nurses, and dietitians in the techniques for teaching self-care of diabetes mellitus. The board accepted the proposal with the stipulation that he find alternative funding for the project within six months.

It took longer than six months, but in July 1967—with the support of the Minnesota Department of Health, the American Diabetes Association, the City of Minneapolis, and the University of Minnesota—the Regional Diabetes Education and Detection Center was launched. The new center was funded by a three-year, $506,000 grant from the U.S. Public Health Service. Etzwiler and E. Bud Cohen served as co-directors and Wyman Jacobson as detection director. St. Louis Park Medical Center provided laboratory support, Asbury Methodist Hospital in downtown Minneapolis provided the necessary space, and the American Rehabilitation Foundation acted as the grant administrator.

The Regional Diabetes Education and Detection Center set four major goals: to provide diabetes-specific education and assistance to professionals in many fields who interact with the individual diabetic; to maintain an outpatient clinic for periodic referrals by physicians; to improve mass-screening techniques; and to do public education on diabetes. The center's first seminar on diabetes for health professionals was held in August 1967.

By 1969, caught in the Nixon era cutbacks in public health funding, the renamed Diabetes Education Center ran out of money. Etzwiler requested and received rent-free space in the basement of the Arneson Building to continue the program. President Norman Sterrie observed in his annual report for 1972 that in "bringing the Diabetes Education Center under our wing . . . we recognized the value of this program for what it has already accomplished and saw in its structure a potential education center for many other areas of medical care."[73] It was from the basement of the Arneson Building that the Diabetes Education Center took on a broader role in patient education for the St. Louis Park Medical Center and that the present International Diabetes Center took shape.

Prior to 1962, diabetic children were most often confined at home, close to their physicians and the emergency rooms they often needed due to improper management of their condition. Camp Needlepoint, organized by the Twin Cities Diabetes Association, gave diabetic children an outdoor camping experience. Donnell Etzwiler was asked in 1962 if he would be interested in the position of camp physician. He responded with a report urging drastic changes in the philosophy of the medical program. Somewhat to his surprise, the association agreed.

"The medical staff at the camp had been distributing urine test bottles, collecting them, doing the test, measuring the dosages, and giving the injections," Etzwiler recalled in 1994. "I thought the kids ought to be doing their own tests, giving their own injections . . . , making learning a priority . . . and increasing their ability to take care of themselves." Camp Needlepoint, Etzwiler noted, provided an ideal laboratory to explore the relationship between patient knowledge, self-care, and outcomes in patients with chronic illnesses.

Clinical Laboratories

St. Louis Park Medical Center clinical laboratories grew rapidly during the 1960s. Leonard Benedict, a Mayo-Clinic-trained biochemist, was hired in 1960 to bring the attention of a full-time scientist to the ever-more complex tests and research the lab was being asked to perform. Wyman Jacobson served as medical director of the lab until his second term as president of St. Louis Park Medical Center began in 1965.

Quality control, always important in a laboratory, was close to an obsession at St. Louis Park. Continuous testing and improvement of techniques allowed Jacobson and Benedict to report to the board in 1961 that the laboratory had matched or exceeded the control limits published by the University Hospital Clinical Laboratory in all ten chemical procedures listed. Working closely with the Methodist Hospital Pathology Laboratory, Benedict achieved "a duplication between our two laboratories almost as good as duplicate determinations which have been assayed in the same laboratory."[74] During the mid-

St. Louis Park Medical Center physicians actively participated in the programs of the Twin Cities Diabetes Association throughout the 1960s. The critical issue for the association at this time was the identification of diabetics. A mobile diabetes detection lab, the first in the United States, was dedicated to this purpose by Wyman Jacobson, then director of the association. Leonard Benedict, supervisor of the medical center laboratory, installed the donated equipment in a converted bus and lent a lab technician, Judy Nelson, to travel with the unit.

1960s, the Social Security Administration and the State of Minnesota established laboratory survey programs to ensure that test results from different labs were reliable and accurate. In 1969, after four years of comparing his test results with those of the other 141 reporting labs, Benedict presented the data, which, he said, warranted the physicians' "unquestioning reliance" on their own lab's accuracy.[75]

Aided by the St. Louis Park Medical Center Research Foundation (see chapter 10), the laboratory department provided regular support for the special research projects carried on by the group. "The extra work and long hours needed to accumulate data and provide the equipment for bacteriologic studies involving several physicians working on different projects," Benedict said of the research work in 1964, "has paid off in providing the general practice . . . with improved methods of collecting and plating specimens."[76] Benedict was elected president of the St. Louis Park Medical Center Research Foundation in 1964, an indication of the important role the laboratory played in stimulating and supporting the group's research programs.

As specialty medicine in the United States became more dependent on a growing range of sophisticated tests, the St. Louis Park Medical Center laboratory aggressively tested new equipment as it became available, selecting the methods best suited to the group's clinical and research needs. In 1967, the department purchased a $32,000 automated twelve-channel blood analyzer in anticipation of the move to the new Northland Building. This was the first of many large capital expenditures to support the basic science of medicine.

An In-House Pharmacy

In April 1960, the medical center moved a step closer to becoming a one-stop health care center with the opening of an in-house pharmacy. Several years of discussion, however, and some controversy had preceded the debut of the Medcenter Pharmacy.

Sponsorship of pharmacies by physician groups had long been deemed unethical and in some cases illegal by the Minnesota Pharmacy Board. While some in the group were sensitive to antagonizing local medical and pharmacy groups, others supported the idea of providing a convenient pharmacy for their patients. Unable to agree, the group set the matter aside until 1958, when newly recruited surgeon Robert Benjamin was put in charge of a committee to investigate the cost of medical supplies. Benjamin, barely six months into his practice at St. Louis Park Medical Center, visited the pharmacies and administrators of the Nicollet Clinic and others to compare the cost savings an affiliated pharmacy could offer. While the cost savings were significant, the real benefit Benjamin believed was in adding a pharmacist to the health care team: "It was a logical thing. . . . It was a convenience for our patients, and it was an opportunity to develop a more sophisticated formulary, in cooperation with a skilled pharmacist."

With approval to continue studying the question granted in the fall of 1958, Benjamin's committee came back with a full proposal in March 1959. "As physicians," he wrote, "we are inextricably involved in the economics in any and all arrangements of drug retailing. We are obligated to continually change our methods and practices so that we conform with the sound professional and economic principles that will provide our patients with the finest health care at the most reasonable cost." The pharmacy, staffed by a specialist in pharmacology, would mean "liberation from hard-sell drug merchandising, pooling of our knowledge of pharmacology, and continual evaluation of our prescription writing habits."[77]

By month's end, the group resolved their qualms about the ethics of on-site drug sales and approved plans to install a small pharmacy office in the south entry lobby. One year later, Ray Anderson, a registered pharmacist, was brought

In 1978, a group of Children's Hospital supporters assembled to celebrate Arnold Anderson's eleven years as medical director and president. Dr. Milton Senn, renowned professor of pediatrics from Yale University, told the group, "Arnold Anderson's personal war was not only against military aggression . . ., but against all misfortunes that befall children, whether ill health, poverty, or racial discrimination. The center that he has created here with you is a living testimony to the faith of Anderson, to the faith of the citizens of this community, faith which transcended the role of chance." [80]

aboard as owner/manager of the Medcenter Pharmacy. The clinic provided the start-up financing, retaining a 49 percent ownership interest. The remaining 51 percent interest was purchased by Ray Anderson.

The small renovation necessary to create the pharmacy was a preview of the major construction projects that would follow in close succession during the 1960s. *Clini Call*, the medical center's in-house newsletter, caught the spirit of the occasion, noting "the pounding hammers, drills and floating sawdust are a small price to pay for the thrill of seeing our new pharmacy emerging from the debris."[78]

ACADEMIC AND COMMUNITY WORK

The creative energy of the founders and other early St. Louis Park Medical Center physicians continued to evolve, often leading them away from the medical center. Some left permanently to pursue academic and leadership challenges not available in private practice. Alvin Schultz started this parade, leaving in 1959 to become chief of medicine at Mt. Sinai Hospital, and then at Hennepin County General Hospital. Don Freeman followed Schultz to General Hospital in 1966 to head the obstetrics and gynecology department. John LaBree became director of medical education at St. Mary's Hospital in Minneapolis in 1970, and William Fifer left the same year to head the Northlands Regional Medical Program at the University of Minnesota, a federally funded program investigating quality, access, and cost control. Richard Webber left the St. Louis Park Medical Center Surgery Department for medical reasons in 1969, regained his health, and went on to help create the SHARE Health Plan.

Arnold Anderson, spiritual leader of the medical center's pediatrics department, was approached by a group of

Minneapolis pediatricians in 1965 with the concept for a children's hospital.[79] He knew the need for operating rooms, laboratories, and other hospital facilities designed for pediatrics. Anderson took a leave of absence from the clinic to organize the medical program for the proposed hospital. Two years later in 1967, he accepted a half-time position as medical director of Children's Hospital of Minneapolis.

In 1967, internist Robert Green accepted the invitation of his friend and former colleague, Alvin Schultz, to organize a new medical tumor clinic in the outpatient department of Hennepin County General Hospital. The tumor clinic that resulted from this collaboration was a multidisciplinary consulting service for General Hospital staff and provided regular in-service instruction on issues relating to the management of cancer. The program, Green said at the time, would "emphasize the total aspects of caring for patients with advanced malignancy, including specific measures of treatment, home care management of the terminal patient, and psychological aspects of advanced malignancy."[81] St. Louis Park Medical Center provided oncology consultations through this program until 1977.

As the medical center settled into its new "ultra-modern" building, another revolution in the delivery of health care was brewing. Matching the turbulent changes in politics, science, and culture, medicine was beginning a vast reorganization based on the experiences of group practices like St. Louis Park Medical Center, the Nicollet Clinic, and the early prepaid medical care plans in the western United States. This emerging trend toward prepaid, comprehensive, health care delivery would profoundly affect the clinic throughout the coming decades.

New attitudes toward family planning and sexuality during the 1960s created a demand for vasectomies, a simple and safe procedure which the majority of doctors were, at the time, unwilling to provide. Robert Benjamin, a surgeon and a firm believer in the right of adults to make their own informed decisions, filled the gap. "I started doing vasectomies in about 1960," Benjamin recalls, "and at that time most of the urologists wouldn't consider doing them."

Things got interesting when a reporter doing a series on the sexual revolution for the Minneapolis Tribune *got Benjamin's name and came to see him. The resulting story, which featured testimonials to the much-improved sex lives of several patients, resulted in jammed phone lines at the St. Louis Park Medical Center. Benjamin set up evening clinics and, with five nurses and one assistant, performed up to twenty procedures each night between 6:00 p.m. and 8:00 p.m.*

9

GROWING UP AND OUT

ST. LOUIS PARK MEDICAL CENTER

1971 TO 1983

By the late 1960s, it was clear to the visionaries within St. Louis Park Medical Center that the bedrock economic structure of medicine was undergoing dramatic change. The cost of medical care, rising in 1969 at a rate nearly two-and-a-half times as fast as the cost of living, was becoming the public's number one worry. Hospital costs were rising even faster, at six times the general cost of living.[82] Local employers, with large commitments to traditional indemnity insurance health benefit plans, were ready to explore alternatives, and the Nixon administration was toying with federal sponsorship of prepaid medicine and the general concepts of the health maintenance organization (HMO). The environment was tailormade for a fast-growing medical group accustomed to charting their own course, a group that had "attracted a critical mass of people who were willing to experiment . . . , to try new procedures, and to look at the delivery of medical care in different ways."[83]

Interest in the development of prepaid medical care first entered the recorded discussions of the medical center in 1961, when President Arnold Anderson suggested that the group "should be ready to work with such plans in the future."[84] Traditional indemnity health insurance plans were limited in the early 1960s to in-hospital care and were largely controlled by and for hospitals. This was creating a serious problem for group practices, which had their own facilities and tended to use hospitals less. "Quite frankly," Anderson told the group in 1963, "unless there is a significant change in health insurance policies in this country, it may become necessary for us to go into the insurance business."[85] In 1964 Anderson urged the group to establish a committee to investigate prepaid insurance. Little progress was made, however, until the building expansion projects of the 1960s were out of the way.

HEALTH PLAN DISCUSSIONS RESURFACE

In 1969 Loren N. Vorlicky, a pediatrician who had joined the group in 1966, revived interest in experimenting with a prepaid medical plan. As chair of the Research and Development Committee, Vorlicky studied existing thought on prepaid medical care and initiated discussions with Interstudy, a Minneapolis think tank, headed by Dr. Paul M. Ellwood. Ellwood at that time was working closely with the Nixon administration to develop federal policies to support the creation of the prepaid group plans he had dubbed "health maintenance organizations." In the spring of 1970, Vorlicky and fellow pediatrician Richard Cushing requested the board's permission to develop a prepaid plan and test its market appeal.

There were several arguments for experimenting with a prepaid health plan. First, as the medical group added outpatient capacity, both in volume and complexity, they were finding it difficult to collect third-party reimbursements for procedures typically done in a hospital, even when the outpatient cost was significantly lower. Third-party insurers, in the late 1960s, believed that treatment in the hospital setting—where there was peer review and established policy—protected them from being "gouged" by physicians. Second, the Twin Cities business community was actively organizing to find ways to hold health insurance costs down, and it seemed likely that the Nixon administration would enact some sort of federal health insurance. With both business and government examining the HMO option, it seemed clear to Vorlicky that the medical center ought to "get some experience operating under a prospective budget."

Vorlicky strongly believed that the clinic's ability to retain its senior physicians lay in its ability to support their academic interests. Prepaid medicine, by stabilizing a portion of the group's income, might allow for a more generous assignment of funds to support teaching and research. A well-run health plan, according to Vorlicky, "was simply a vehicle for the clinic to manage its own future. . . . it was a way for the clinic to grow, manage its resources, develop its referral relationships, stabilize and grow its patient base so it could answer the question: Where is the future business going to come from and how are we going to get paid for it?"

The health maintenance organization is a method of providing comprehensive health care in which patients pay a regular, set fee not related to their use of the system. In return, the HMO promises to provide all necessary medical care and assumes the financial risk. Traditionally, preventative care has been included in an attempt to identify health problems earlier, thereby lowering overall costs to the HMO. There are three types of HMOs: Staff Model HMO; Group Practice Model HMO; and Network Model HMO or Independent Practice Association.

COMPREHENSIVE HEALTH CARE COMMITTEE

Accepting Vorlicky and Cushing's proposal, the board created the Comprehensive Health Care Committee. The board's seriousness about what was then regarded as a "valid social experiment"[86] can be inferred from the roster of the committee, which included Vorlicky, Cushing, Arnold Anderson, Robert Green, and Norman Sterrie. Throughout the remainder of 1970, the committee met with individuals and groups involved in prepaid plans, including Paul Ellwood, Maurice McKay of Group Health of Minnesota, and William Shearer, administrator of the Ross-Loos Clinic in Los Angeles, the oldest and largest physician-run prepaid group practice in the country.

After the health plan was developed, the committee had no great difficulty selling it to the board. The skeptics in the group were comfortable with the idea as a limited experiment and trusted the committee. Existing contacts with employers such as General Mills, Honeywell, and Target Stores allowed committee members to broach the subject of the proposed prepaid health plan with their most important market. There was, Vorlicky reported in early 1971, "increasing enthusiasm on the part of employer groups within our service area to develop or obtain a prepaid health care option for their employee groups."[87]

Next came the task of finding an insurance partner. "Larry [Vorlicky] and I made several trips talking to various companies such as Prudential, Northwestern National Life, and the St. Paul Companies," Norman Sterrie recalled. "It was all very new and we didn't have a lot of statistics, but we did know that one child with a brain tumor could kill the system." By spring of 1971, the committee had settled on a discounted fee-for-service plan operated jointly by the clinic and the St. Paul Companies, which would handle all marketing and would assume all the risk—including the hospital risk. Only after the agreement was signed did the medical center realize that the organization that took the risk also had access to the financial rewards of prepayment. As luck would have it, Minnesota's attorney general held up approval of the plan beyond the 120-day letter of intent between the St. Paul Companies and the medical center, and the plan was dropped.

The committee went back to the drawing board. Interstudy, which received a federal grant to set up a group-practice HMO, lent Richard Burke to help prepare a request for proposals that spelled out the insurance services needed to support a prepaid plan controlled entirely by the medical center. The benefit package, which had been developed in cooperation with General Mill's personnel department, remained the same, but the risk of hospitalization would be shared by the health plan and the insurer. Initial responses from employers were overwhelmingly positive.

MEDCENTER HEALTH PLAN

In April 1972, the St. Louis Park Medical Center Board approved the new plan presented by Vorlicky, Burke, and the Comprehensive Health Care Committee. A nonprofit organization would be created to manage the prepaid plan which was named "Medcenter Health Plan." Northwestern National Life, the company that had most aggressively responded to the clinic's request for proposals, would provide marketing, reinsurance, and technical services on a contract basis.

Initially, the plan would be limited to 5,000 members and would enroll the employees of St. Louis Park Medical Center and Interstudy first. The basic premium for a family of three was set at $61 per month and included all medical and surgical care, hospital coverage, and prescription-drug coverage. The medical center would further support the new health plan by guaranteeing a line of operating credit of up to $75,000.[88] The plan began enrolling patients in November 1972 and by February 1973 had signed up 1,300 members, primarily employees of Pillsbury and Northwestern National Life.

The timing could not have been better. In 1972, the business community had formed and financed a health-care working group, the Twin Cities Health Care Development Project, which was actively advocating for alternatives to traditional health insurance. The local market was moving toward HMO-type solutions, and Medcenter Health Plan was able to begin marketing several months to a year before the Nicollet-Eitel Family Health Plan or other competing prepaid plans got underway.

The new source of patients and revenue came at an important time for the medical center, which was being squeezed between its high debt load from the Northland construction, a collapse in its growth rate, and the price controls President Richard Nixon instituted in August 1971. Once again, the group's willingness to try something new

MEDCENTER HEALTH PLAN FOUNDING BOARD, 1972

Loren Vorlicky, M.D., President
Henry T. Smith, M.D., Vice President
J. Roland Pavek, M.D., Secretary/Treasurer
David Buran, M.D.
Robert Green, M.D.
Walter Indeck, M.D.
Harley Racer, M.D.
Norman Sterrie, M.D.

and to test a new strategy for health care delivery served the long-term interests of the medical center and positioned it to make the most of the changes to come.

A PRIMARY CARE NETWORK

For surgeon Glen D. Nelson, who became a partner in 1969 and was president of St. Louis Park Medical Center from 1975 to 1983, steady growth of the patient base was absolutely indispensable for successful group practice. "The primary goal for which growth was the solution," Nelson said in 1994, "was the ability to attract a critical mass of patients which in turn gave us the capacity to support specialists and subspecialists, who I viewed as the real catalysts for better care and the educators of everyone in the group."

Creating a network of provider groups to whom primary care responsibilities were contracted for a set, or capitated, fee, fit perfectly into Nelson's philosophy of growth. There was simply no faster way to expand the group's patient base to support their growing roster of specialists. The larger patient base would require an extensive system of primary care clinics to provide the majority of day-to-day care and convenient access over a broad geographic region. It was clear that the medical center lacked the resources to build its own primary care network in a reasonable time frame without reducing its support for the specialty and subspecialty departments that were the heart of the group's self-identity. Understanding this, Medcenter administrators Richard Burke and Steve Goldstone proposed in late 1973 that the health plan create a primary care network of the "highest quality medical care groups."[89]

The Medcenter Health Plan negotiated its first primary-care provider contract with the Coon Rapids Clinic in April 1974. The fifteen physician-members of the clinic agreed to provide accessible primary care to Medcenter Health Plan members in the fast-growing northern suburbs. St. Louis Park Medical Center would provide specialty services for a share of the capitation payment, and Mercy Hospital in Coon Rapids would provide hospital care.

The network model worked so well in Coon Rapids that Medcenter Health Plan brought another group to the medical center for approval in 1975. The East Side Comprehensive Health Organization (ECHO), an informal network of family care physicians in East St. Paul, was accepted as a network provider group in January 1976. The twenty-three ECHO physicians were affiliated with St. John's Hospital in St. Paul, and the ready-made network gave Medcenter an immediate presence in the east metro area, home to 3M Company and other major employers.

The pressure to expand the network was not coming solely from within Medcenter Health Plan. In 1975, the Shakopee Medical Center expressed interest in joining Medcenter as a provider group. With six family practice physicians and a general surgeon, the Shakopee group were young, aggressive, and interested in growth. As primary care providers to employees of Toro, Peavey, Cargill, and other major employers, Shakopee had institutional connections that would be helpful in marketing the plan in the south metro area.

By 1977, with the Shakopee clinic in the network, Medcenter Health Plan had grown to 18,000 subscribers. In 1978 it reported 32,000 members, 8,000 of whom had chosen a network provider for their primary care. The network model was a success. Over the next several years, other clinics, such as Gorman Clinic and Woodbury Family Medical Center, were added through the ECHO affiliation.[90]

SATELLITE CLINICS

The network of primary care providers provided access to the Medcenter Health Plan where high-quality groups already existed. In other areas, St. Louis Park Medical Center began to build its own primary care satellites. These were smaller, more intimate "offices where people are used to coming" for primary care services and "where the practitioners are comfortable," according to A. Stuart Hanson, St. Louis Park Medical Center's medical director from 1975 to 1982. "We looked at other models around the country and those who were satelliting had continued to grow. Those that didn't satellite got boxed in." According to Norman Sterrie, the development of satellite offices was key to establishing a tangible link to patients in the far-flung suburbs. "You've got to have an awfully big attraction to get people to come from a long distance," Sterrie said in 1994, "and the way the city was growing, it was apparent to me you had to be where the people are."

Opening satellite offices was not an entirely new idea to St. Louis Park Medical Center. As early as 1964, surgeons Richard Webber and Jerome Grismer had proposed a satellite office adjacent to the new Fairview Southdale Hospital. Theirs was an idea ahead of its time, and it was dropped by the board. By 1971, however, President Norman Sterrie had revived interest in the concept and created the Satellite Committee under the leadership of a young physician, Edward Kraus. Kraus and his committee began serious consideration of satellite options in late 1971.[91]

One thing Sterrie did not want to do was antagonize suburban physicians whose referrals made up a small but important percentage of the medical center's practice. He had Roger Asplin study the demographics of the surrounding suburbs, looking for communities with few or no physicians. The community of Plymouth was underserved at the time and was close to General Mills, a long-time supporter of the medical center and one of the corporations leading the Twin Cities Health Care Development Project. When the Plymouth satellite office opened in September 1972[92] at the corner of Interstate 494 and Highway 55, it was just a stone's throw from Betty Crocker's kitchen.

The results after less than one year were encouraging. "Our growth in Plymouth has exceeded all projections," Norman Sterrie wrote in his 1972 annual report. Happy with the results, the board approved the addition of two more satellite offices. In August 1974, the "Minnetonka" office opened in the Christy Building at the corner of Highways 101 and 7 under the leadership of family physician Donald Pine. In January 1975, the office of general practitioner Floyd Swenson, located near the Ridgedale Shopping Center in Minnetonka, joined the medical center's satellite system.[93]

This rapid expansion into the western suburbs, while well timed to meet the needs of the growing Medcenter Health Plan, had not previously been part of a long-term plan. The immediate problem was finding enough qualified primary care doctors to staff the rapidly growing satellites. No additional offices were approved in 1975, although planning continued in an effort to meet the "intense community demand" for sites in the south suburbs, Hopkins, and downtown.[94]

St. Louis Park Medical Center had a tradition of assigning young physicians—fresh from residency training—either an academic or a practice-based project. Internist Edward Kraus, for example, started at the clinic in July 1971. Less than six months later he was leading the committee to find and develop the medical center's first satellite clinic.

GEOGRAPHIC EXPANSION

As the Medcenter Health Plan continued to grow, it exerted more influence on the medical center's decision making. Throughout 1976 Steve Goldstone, who had succeeded Richard Burke as Medcenter Health Plan executive director, argued for the development of a satellite in the south suburbs where the Nicollet Clinic had been since 1971, but staff and capital shortages at the existing offices dictated other priorities. In mid-1976, the St. Louis Park Medical Center Board authorized the purchase of land along Highways 101 and 7 for the construction of new space for the Minnetonka office. Plans included space for a Medcenter pharmacy, Benson Optical, and at least five dentists. Lacking sufficient internal financing for capital expansion, a group of medical center physicians and a dentistry group formed a limited partnership, the Minnetonka Physicians and Dentists Building Associates, to finance construction. Donald Pine moved his staff of primary care physicians into the new building in August 1977.

A new satellite in Hopkins opened in leased space in April 1977. Like the Plymouth clinic organized by Ed Kraus and the primary care offices of the Nicollet Clinic, the Hopkins office was staffed by physicians from the traditional primary care specialties—internal medicine, pediatrics, and obstetrics and gynecology.

Finding financing for office construction helped to put the brakes on geographic expansion. Medcenter Health Plan, anxious to expand its presence in the rapidly growing southern suburbs, offered to help finance a satellite in the Burnsville area in late 1977. The St. Louis Park Medical Center Board, however, was more interested in developing other areas first. Another clinic, staffed along the lines of the Hopkins clinic and headed by Ed Kraus, opened in Bloomington in 1978. The Bloomington office grew rapidly and in 1982 moved to a new, larger site in a renovated theater. It continues to use physicians trained in the traditional primary care specialties to provide services that family practice physicians provide in other satellite clinics.

Construction of a new office in Plymouth began in August 1979. General contractor M. A. Mortenson partnered with the medical center in the development of this project, helping to alleviate the need to find scarce and high-priced construction loan money. Another project, in the suburb of Brooklyn Center, was seriously considered between 1978 and 1981 at the request of the Medcenter Health Plan, but the details could not be worked out.

In August 1979 St. Louis Park Medical Center secured a satellite site in downtown Minneapolis with the addition of internist Markle Karlen. His small office adjacent to the downtown Metropolitan Medical Center (MMC), the former Swedish and St. Barnabas hospitals, became a general internal medicine office and a base for subspecialists working at the MMC.[95] Another hospital-based subspecialty office opened in the Meadowbrook Building adjacent to Methodist Hospital to house the neurology department and provide a convenient suite of offices for the hospital-based obstetricians. This first of several Meadowbrook offices opened in early 1982.

By late 1982, the arguments for a new office in the Burnsville/Eagan area became impossible to ignore. Medcenter Health Plan, now accounting for more than 54 percent of St. Louis Park Medical Center's activity, was anxious enough for a primary care facility in this area to guarantee capitation for four thousand patients in the first year. With these assurances from the health plan, the medical center opened the new Eagan satellite only a few miles from the Nicollet Clinic Eagan office. Pediatrician Theresa A. Ryan served as site leader and host of the ribbon-cutting ceremony in July 1982, attended by Minnesota Governor Al Quie.

Although the Nicollet Clinic had been first to begin creating a satellite network, the much larger St. Louis Park Medical Center quickly got out in front in the western suburbs. Only in the Burnsville/Eagan area did the Nicollet Clinic retain a solid lead through the 1970s. By the time the two groups decided to merge in 1983, St. Louis Park Medical Center was operating six, primary-care metro-area satellites, while the Nicollet Clinic was operating four.

The steady growth of the satellite system at St. Louis Park Medical Center had few opponents, but it wasn't without pain. Founder George Lund, for instance, remembers the pain of realizing his patients were choosing the access and convenience of the satellite offices over their personal relationships to a long-time physician. "I was hurt that people could be so fickle, that I wasn't important to them . . . ," he recalls, adding that even at the time he realized that "I had put myself on a level on which I didn't belong."

NORTHLAND CAMPUS EXPANDS

Rapid growth in the early 1970s pushed the limits of existing space in the Northland Building. Renovation to create new space to house departments that had remained in the Arneson Building began in 1972. Ophthalmology, for instance, moved to the second floor of the Northland Building in 1973, allowing for critical expansion of the HMO staff and the family practice residency program in

As was the case in the construction of the Northland Building, physicians and staff collaborated with the architect and builder on the renovation of the building. This process resulted in a unique layout for the ophthalmology examining rooms. To create the distance of 18 feet needed for eye exams, the architect placed tunnels side by side between two adjoining opthalmology rooms, which were approached from opposite ends. The result was two private examining rooms in just over half the previous space required for one examining room.

the Arneson Building. Pediatrics moved to the first basement, or ground level, of the Northland Building. During this time the shelled-in sixth floor was also finished. By 1974, a sluggish economy and high debt load forced President Norman Sterrie to call a halt to any construction beyond what was absolutely necessary.

After two more years of dramatic growth, expansion of the Northland Building was taken up again in 1976, this time under the leadership of Glen Nelson and Tom Dunkel, chair of the Building Committee. With architect Jack Wilwerding of Setter, Leach & Lindstrom, Inc., the committee planned a two-story addition to the north side of the existing building. It would house the allergy, family practice, oncology, and neurology departments, as well as provide new space for the expanded medical records and computer departments. At $2.5 million the addition "cost about the same as the first seven floors of the Northland Building," according to Roger Asplin. In 1977, the group again honored Morton and Katheren Arneson, their original benefactors, by naming the completed structure "the Arneson Pavillion."

WORKING WITH METHODIST

From the day it opened in 1959, Methodist Hospital was an important part of the growth and success of St. Louis Park Medical Center. The hospital provided the group with state-of-the art inpatient medical facilities within minutes of their own offices. The medical center was no less important to the hospital, providing a large, ready-made base of patients, an excellent medical reputation, and an academically motivated group willing to work to upgrade the overall level of hospital services.

St. Louis Park Medical Center physicians had been consulted early in the planning process for Methodist Hospital and had been welcomed by the hospital administration from the beginning. But a modern hospital is a complex political environment. Almost immediately after the hospital opened, medical center physicians found themselves engaged in a quiet three-way struggle with the hospital administration and the independent physicians. The independent medical staff—the physicians practicing on their own and in small partnerships—were anxious to see the hospital protect their rights of access against St. Louis Park Medical Center, which was growing rapidly and openly challenging many of the long-held notions of private practice. To curb the largest group practicing in the new hospital, the nonclinic majority added provisions to the hospital medical staff bylaws to prevent medical center physicians from succeeding each other as department heads or from having more than one member serve as an officer of the medical staff. According to Wyman Jacobson, who served several terms as St. Louis Park Medical Center president during this period, the hospital eventually ran out of nonclinic physicians who were willing to serve and subsequently removed these provisions from the bylaws. The tradition, however, of alternating between clinic and nonclinic leadership has been informally carried forward to the present.

Despite the underlying tensions, the medical center's contributions continued to grow. By the late 1960s, St. Louis Park Medical Center was performing 55 percent of the surgeries at Methodist Hospital. The Artificial Kidney Center at the hospital had been created by Donald Duncan. Other medical center physicians—Charles L. Murray, John H. Brown, Robert Green, and Loren Vorlicky—were instrumental in developing the Methodist Hospital oncology programs in the early 1970s. Virtually all of the specialty conferences during the 1960s and 1970s were sponsored by St. Louis Park Medical Center physicians, and both the surgery and the family practice residency programs were started at the hospital during this period by St. Louis Park Medical Center physicians.

For almost a decade the tensions were allowed to fester. Hospital administrators Vernon Spry and Earl Dresser were determined to avoid even the appearance of a special relationship between the medical center and the hospital. In the mid-1960s, the steadily increasing interdependence of the two organizations made the establishment of some degree of formal relations necessary, so Wyman Jacobson and Earl Young began a series of conversations with Dresser to try to create a better working relationship.

"Staff relations were dismal," said Norman Sterrie, recalling the period shortly after he became president of St. Louis Park Medical Center in 1970. "I started meeting with Earl [Dresser] very early with the feeling that medicine is a total thing and we were both big contributors to the whole." By 1971, he reported "warmer hospital relationships" and proposed that the group should "go more than half way" in their efforts to "achieve a strong hospital base."[96]

Relations continued to improve. In 1973, Glen Nelson implemented an arrangement to provide St. Louis Park Medical Center-staffed emergency services at Methodist Hospital for St. Louis Park Medical Center patients. Nelson reported that "an excellent working relationship with Methodist" had been established, "allowing the Medical Center to provide 24 hour coverage for its HMO patients within the confines of our group."[97]

New efforts at cooperation did not, however, extend to the development of a regional system of satellite clinics in 1971 or the Medcenter Health Plan in 1972. During the development of these new delivery systems the arms-length relationship "really hurt us as far as trying to develop a comprehensive health care organization," according to Robert Benjamin, referring to the opportunities that might have been seized if the financial resources of the hospital could have been strategically combined with the energy of the medical center.

The mutual dependence continued to increase. With more than 120 physicians, the medical center was responsible for an increasing percentage of hospital revenues. The Medcenter Health Plan alone accounted for 20 percent of the surgeries performed there, and the medical center routinely counted on Methodist for 80 percent of its inpatient medical care.

Late in 1981, the two organizations agreed to jointly hire business consultants Booz, Allen and Hamilton to "identify areas of common purpose and help work out the communications problems."[98] The firm's recommendations—including the development of shared or overlapping governance, the joint planning of activities, and on-going management coordination and communication—were politely received. A proposal to exchange board members in an ex-officio capacity was implemented in June 1982 when Earl Dresser began attending board meetings of the St. Louis Park Medical Center. President Glen Nelson, in turn, began attending board meetings at Methodist Hospital.

URGENT CARE CENTER, INC.

A project was needed to test the new spirit of cooperation. St. Louis Park Medical Center approached Methodist Hospital with the idea of establishing a for-profit "Urgent Care Center." The fact that the Nicollet Clinic had just announced that its new "Urgicenter" would open on July 6, 1982, added urgency to the idea.

By September, the hospital and the medical center had hammered out the details of the new project, and the results reveal a good deal about the tensions that remained. In spite of the fact that the Urgent Care Center was technically an ambulatory medical facility, the hospital refused to accept a subordinate position in its management or to allow the medical center to manage the delivery of care in a manner consistent with the care provided to its other patients. Methodist insisted that patient medical records be kept separate from St. Louis Park Medical Center patient records and that the Urgent Care Center be publicly identified as a service affiliate of Methodist Hospital. The St. Louis Park Medical Center Board considered these "disadvantages" but concluded that the experience of operating a joint project with the hospital outweighed the negatives.[99]

The jointly owned Urgent Care Center opened in February 1983 in the medical center's Ridgedale office. Ownership in the new organization was shared equally by the hospital and the clinic. Professional staffing was contracted to St. Louis Park Medical Center and the Emergency Physicians Professional Association (EPPA), which had by this time also taken over emergency room duties for St. Louis Park Medical Center at Methodist Hospital. The first small steps toward the joint planning and governance Booz Allen envisioned had been taken. Further steps toward affiliation would have to wait.

The race between the medical center and Nicollet Clinic to implement the urgent care idea was just one indication that the two were beginning to compete directly. In 1982 St. Louis Park Medical Center moved its Ridgedale primary care satellite to a new office across the street from the Nicollet Clinic's Ridgedale satellite, which had opened less than a month earlier. That same year, St. Louis Park Medical Center opened a new satellite in Eagan, one year after the Nicollet Clinic had done the same. The Nicollet-Eitel Health Plan, in need of more young, suburban families to balance its urban base, was aggressively discounting its premiums for large corporate groups, like Control Data, and was successfully luring patients away from the larger Medcenter Health Plan and Group Health. Both clinics were nearing the limits of their ability to grow internally and both were keenly aware that a safe haven would not be available during the coming shakeout in the Twin Cities health care market. It would only be a matter of time before talk of merging the two group practices would begin in earnest.

10

CONTINUING THE COMMITMENT

RESEARCH AND EDUCATION

The commitment of the founders to education and research, articulated by Robert Green in 1958 and cast in bronze for all to see, was given organizational life in July 1959 with the incorporation of the St. Louis Park Medical Center Research Foundation. Not limited to supporting the activities of the center's physicians, the foundation was dedicated to "the task of restoring to the whole community of physicians the attitudes of scholarship and self-evaluation so often sacrificed to the complexity of modern practice."[100]

Arnold Anderson was the first to recognize the need for financial separation between medical center operations and research and education activities. Having received a small amount of outside income from the Washburn Memorial Clinic for his work with brain-injured children, Anderson needed a place to put the funds where they could be reserved for future research work. With the help of attorney William Green, the tax-exempt St. Louis Park Medical Center Research Foundation was created to provide an administrative structure, technical aid, and a forum for review to support and stimulate creative energy both within and outside of the medical center. George Lund credited Anderson for bringing the foundation into existence: "It was a great idea. . . . It gave [our education and

ST. LOUIS PARK MEDICAL CENTER RESEARCH FOUNDATION FOUNDING BOARD, 1959

Arnold Anderson, M.D., President
Jerome Grismer, M.D., Vice President
William Green, Attorney, Secretary
James Harris, Northwestern National Bank, Treasurer
Roger Asplin, Executive Secretary
David Babcock, Dayton's
William Fifer, M.D.
Walter Indeck, M.D.
George Lund, M.D.
Jack A. Vennes, M.D.

research programs] a focus and an organizational structure, as well as a place of accountability."

FIRST MEDICAL CONFERENCE

Mead Johnson Corporation gave one of the first gifts to the new foundation to support Anderson's work in cerebral dysfunction in children. Anderson had proposed bringing a group of educators, physicians, parents, and researchers together to "determine whether or not a grass roots, interdisciplinary exchange . . . can discover and develop methods and resources which will improve the understanding and treatment of . . . the child with cerebral dysfunction."[101] It was a fresh, collegial approach to a serious community problem and modeled after the multidisciplinary, collaborative approach to medical problems that prevailed within the medical center. The Cerebral Dysfunction Conference, held in January 1961 and cosponsored by the Richfield Public Schools, was enthusiastically received by the participants. The booklet of the proceedings, prepared by the foundation, was in its third printing by 1964.

The success of the Cerebral Dysfunction Conference demonstrated the benefits of the multidisciplinary approach to community health and education problems. It also demonstrated to St. Louis Park Medical Center the important service the foundation could provide in creating a charitable link with the community. "If we had attempted to sponsor such a project through [the medical group] in 1961," Anderson told the annual meeting in 1964, "community resistance would have killed it, yet there was no other pediatric group in our community that had the vision or organization to sponsor such a project. The foundation stepped in and provided the needed sponsorship." He went on to predict that the foundation would "play an ever-increasing role in our total medical service."[102]

ESTABLISHING A BASE

The foundation's growing role was made possible, in part, by financial support from the medical center. This support started in 1961 when $1,000, approximately 5 percent of that year's profit, was donated. By 1971, the medical center's annual donation had grown to $20,000.

The 1960s were a time of tremendous activity and growth for the foundation. It gave small grants or administrative support to research projects ranging from Robert Benjamin's "On-going study of gall bladder disease," to Donnell Etzwiler's "Study on education of children regarding their disease," to the "Study of the efficiency of the para-cervical block as a delivery anesthesia," by Donald Freeman, Alex Barno, and Melvin Baken Jr. The medical library, located in the lower level of the Arneson Building and newly redecorated as a gift from Morten Arneson, became a symbol of the group's commitment to supporting continuing education and medical research. This unique asset was transferred to the foundation in 1963.

In 1962, Anderson turned over leadership of the foundation to thoracic surgeon, Jerome Grismer. Leonard Benedict, head of the St. Louis Park Medical Center laboratory, was then elected foundation president in 1964. By 1968 the volume and variety of the research and education projects had grown enough to require formal coordination beyond the scope of these volunteer leadership positions. William Fifer suggested that a physician working half-time could significantly improve research and education efforts and requested the position for himself. The medical center board approved the request in 1969, freeing Fifer to become the foundation's first director of medical education, responsible to both the clinic and the foundation. Fifer's plan for the foundation called for the creation of the intellectual climate needed to press forward with initiatives "to enhance the comprehensiveness of medical care."[103]

"It is with humility that we of the St. Louis Park Medical Foundation set ourselves to the task of developing an organization for the purpose of fostering research and teaching. . . . Our own experience . . . has demonstrated to us that if the public is to enjoy the full service potential of medicine, teaching and research at some level must also become an integral part of the professional life of the physician whose principal role is the practice of medicine among families in a community."

St. Louis Park Medical Center Research Foundation Prospectus, *1963*

GROWTH DURING THE 1970S

Under the quiet leadership of Fifer and pediatrician Don Amren, elected president in 1972, the foundation continued to grow. Elaine Anderson, a former business school teacher who had worked with Arnold Anderson on the Cerebral Dysfunction Conference, was employed half-time to help with fund-raising efforts and to provide administrative support. In 1969, the foundation distributed $38,000 to fund the education and medical research efforts of clinic physicians. By 1975, this amount had risen to $83,500, a significant proportion of which was raised by asking professional-courtesy patients to voluntarily give their insurance reimbursements to the foundation.[104] Of that amount, $51,000 was administered as pass-through grants from other sources. The balance was raised from a growing membership list recruited from the physicians, staff, and patient community.

As the foundation grew, it became increasingly valuable to the larger medical community as well as to the clinic. At the instigation of cardiologist Charles Peterson, the foundation funded its first medical education seminar entitled "Correlative Electrocardiology for the Primary Care Physician." Held in June 1973 at Breezy Point Lodge in northern Minnesota, the program attracted thirty-six physicians and was considered successful enough that a regular schedule of seminars was planned. Elaine Anderson served as seminar coordinator. By 1978, the foundation was sponsoring four or five two-day accredited seminars each year. The seminar program continued to grow in popularity, attracting more than 500 physicians and 250 other health professionals to six seminars in 1984.[105] The professional education program is still in operation today.

TRANSFERRING ASSETS

As the medical center's financial situation improved through 1974, President Norman Sterrie initiated a strategy to address several problems related to owning increasingly valuable real estate and medical facilities. More than ten years earlier, Arnold Anderson, Richard Webber, and Roger Asplin had made a trip to the Ocshner Clinic in New Orleans to investigate the possibility of transferring clinic properties to the research foundation. In his annual report for 1963, Anderson told the group, "The visit increased our awareness of the fact that as hospitals extend their outpatient services, their tax advantages will become an increasingly serious problem for us."[106] Comparison of operating data of the country's larger group medical clinics in 1974 revealed St. Louis Park Medical Center to have one of the lowest expense ratios, yet it was facing the highest property tax expense of any of the clinics in the survey.[107] Area hospitals, as nonprofit charities, were not paying property taxes on their facilities, nor were they liable for taxes on income in excess of expenses, which they could then reinvest in the hospital infrastructure. The transfer, which was rejected as premature in the 1960s, was put back on the agenda by Sterrie. Although the medical center had not declared a profit since the construction of the Northland Building in 1968, profitability was returning in the mid-1970s. This was a happy result, but one which also carried negative tax consequences.

The tax problems were serious enough, but there was another more immediate problem. The growing value of the properties was putting the goal of equal ownership out of reach for new physicians. Internist A. Stuart Hanson, who joined the group in 1971, recalled, "I had an opportunity, after I'd been there a year, to buy into Medcenter, Inc., for $34,000, which happened to be the exact amount I had just paid for my house. I was going to have to borrow the whole amount . . . which would have taken all my disposable income." Roger Asplin worried at the time that the value of the shareholders stock in the property company was rising beyond the ability of the group to buy back the shares of retiring physicians, which would jeopardize the ability of the group to maintain control of all the shares.

"I was as big an owner as anyone," Robert Benjamin stated in 1994, "but it wasn't good for morale to have some people who owned the buildings collecting their rent every month . . . and the others not owning. We knew it wasn't right." Norman Sterrie believed that a system was needed "to get rid of the properties in a way that we wouldn't have a last man's club owning all the properties." The solution was a transfer of the property assets from the property corporation to the nonprofit foundation.

Roger Asplin and counsel D. James Nielson worked out the details of the transfer over a four-year period. "What we decided," Asplin said, "was to have the doctors contribute half the appreciated value of their stocks in Medcenter, Inc., to the foundation. The foundation then bought the other half with money raised through a bond sale. The bonds were paid off out of the rental paid by the medical center to the foundation for the use of the buildings." The gift to the foundation could be used to reduce the capital gains taxes owed on the appreciated value of the property shares, and the gift would provide a reliable source of income to the foundation after the bonds were paid off.

After selling $1.5 million in bonds, the foundation acquired all of the shares in Medcenter, Inc., by December 1975. "It was an equity issue," noted Glen Nelson, who was president of the medical center when the transfer was completed. "It provided a return on an appreciated investment for the then-current owners and at the same time obviated the potential conflict that would grow over time with the differential ownership among the physicians in the group."[108] The net result was a transfer of a $6-million asset to the foundation, providing a solid base to, as Roger Asplin put it, "support significantly more programs of medical education and research."[109]

COMING OF AGE IN THE 1980S

The gift-sale of building assets to the foundation in 1975 put the foundation in a position to assume a major role in the development of the medical center. The *Bulletin*, the medical center's quarterly publication and long a source of pride within the group, was transferred to the foundation in 1976, along with a pledge of $10,000 per year to support its publication. Clinic Administrator Roger Asplin managed the foundation on an unpaid basis until 1979 when he became the foundation's first full-time executive director. When Asplin retired in 1982, pediatrician Paul Batalden, who became foundation president in 1981, honored him as "the architect and prime mover of the foundation. We cannot adequately express our admiration for Mr. Asplin's many accomplishments, his unwavering faith in the foundation's mission, his pioneering spirit, his professionalism, and his generous support."[110]

Faced with Asplin's impending retirement, the foundation board offered the position of executive director to James V. Toscano, a manager with a wealth of experience in the nonprofit arts and media world. Then president of the Minnesota Museum of American Art, Toscano was intimately familiar with the challenges of raising financial support from the philanthropic community in the Twin Cities and had demonstrated the ability to put together complex multiorganization agreements involving real estate, finance, and marketing. Executive director was not a position the leadership of the foundation took lightly. Toscano's qualifications and attitudes were intensely scrutinized by the search committee and the board. "I was recruited here in the spring of 1981, largely on the recommendation of Jim Shannon, who was then the head of the General Mills Foundation . . . and five months later I was hired," Toscano said. "It was the longest process I had ever been through."

With substantial assets, a reliable source of income, and a growing professional staff, the foundation began to assert its role as the long-term repository of the good ideas and humanitarian projects initiated by the physicians and staff of the medical center. The most significant of these in terms of the growth and development of the foundation was St. Louis Park Medical Center's Quality Assurance Program (see chapter 11). The Health Services Research Center was created within the foundation in 1976 to manage and expand this program after its initial success. The Quality Assurance Program was the first of several large projects started within the medical center as individual projects that were later incorporated into the nonprofit mission of the foundation.

TACKLING CHRONIC DISEASE: DIABETES

Less than a year after the Health Services Research Center was incorporated into the foundation, the Diabetes Education Center was also brought under its wing. Started in the mid-1960s by pediatrician Donnell Etzwiler, the diabetes center reflected Etzwiler's belief in a team approach to chronic disease care in which the patient plays the central role. This belief was successfully translated into practice in the education and care provided by the diabetes center, but attempts in the early 1970s to fulfill Etzwiler's vision of extending the diabetes model to other chronic diseases did not fare as well because of difficulty in raising funds.

In 1973, a time when patient education was a relatively new concept, the center hosted a three-day conference entitled "Educating the Patient with Diabetes." Being among the first to recognize the importance of patient knowledge and participation in chronic disease care, the center was recognized in 1975 with a grant from the McKnight Foundation to work in cooperation with the Minnesota affiliate of the American Diabetes Association

(ADA) to bring diabetes education to patients around the state. The TEAM program sent a physician/nurse/dietitian team into fifty-two communities that year to present a one-and-a-half-day workshop for health professionals and patients focusing on the importance of diabetes education in diabetes care.

"Quality, comprehensive health care requires informed patients cooperating with knowledgeable and concerned health professionals in a planned system of management."

Donnell Etzwiler, M.D.

The TEAM workshops were complemented by a five-day intensive training program that had been started at the center some years before. In 1978, 417 patients and 323 health professionals went through the program. By 1980, more than 4,500 patients and 3,500 health professionals had completed the five-day training, which by then was scheduled every other week in the cramped diabetes education facilities in the basement of the Arneson Building.[111] This program is still in operation today, attracting patients, health professionals, and industry professionals alike.

The center's core work in diabetes care and education was aided by Etzwiler's growing national prominence in the field. Etzwiler chaired the Treatment Committee of the National Commission on Diabetes in 1975 and served as president of the American Diabetes Association in 1976, a position that required 120 days of special leave time from the pediatrics department and "a significant sacrifice on the part of my colleagues," he said.

Etzwiler was also involved with Camp Needlepoint, a diabetes camp for children. Many diabetes camps, then and now, were associated with state ADA affiliates. Recognizing the need for updating the camp programs, Etzwiler and the Diabetes Education Center organized the first international workshop on diabetes and camping in 1974. Health professionals from around the country and the world participated in the program, coming together to share ideas and to discuss ways to improve the camps. The proceedings were published and the group continued to meet annually, eventually leading to the establishment of standards and accreditation for camps through the ADA.

In 1977, the Minnesota Department of Health contracted with the foundation and the Diabetes Education Center to conduct a statewide health education program. Called the Health Education for Living Program (HELP), it was the first comprehensive, statewide patient education program in the country. By 1979, the program, funded in part by the McKnight Foundation and coordinated by Carelyn Fylling, M.S., R.N., had reached sixty-eight Minnesota communities.

International Diabetes Center

After several years of rapid growth, the Diabetes Education Center needed new space. Russell Ewald, then executive director of the McKnight Foundation, was interested in the idea of a model for chronic care and suggested that the center was a project worthy of a major capital campaign. After seeing the cramped space in which the center was operating, Ewald suggested that "we talk to someone in construction to see what a world-class diabetes center would cost," said Etzwiler.

With the interest of the McKnight Foundation aroused, it fell to James Toscano and a consultant, Andrew Curry, to develop a capital campaign the McKnight Foundation could support. "I was brought in, in part, to help conceptualize [the diabetes center], to interpret it," explained Toscano. In the process, "we renamed it. We called it the International Diabetes Center and, clearly, some thought the name was presumptuous. But we had an international reputation and international ties, so I said, 'Let's go with it.'" The architectural firm that had designed the original Northland Building, Setter, Leach & Lindstrom, Inc., was asked to design a building to meet the needs of the proposed International Diabetes Center. The firm's design, a four-story building, was estimated to cost $7.5 million.

Over several months, the development team of Etzwiler, Toscano, Curry, and William Henry, then administrator of the new International Diabetes Center, prepared a detailed proposal for the McKnight Foundation. As primary funders, McKnight agreed to contribute $5 million. St. Louis Park Medical Center was to raise the remaining $2.5 million from the staff and the community to complete the project. Glen Nelson signaled the medical center's full support for the project when he agreed to head the fund-raising committee. Dale Olseth, president of Medtronic, Inc., was co-chair of the committee, which also included Elmer L. Anderson, former governor and chairman of H. B. Fuller, Inc.; L. D. DeSimone, executive vice president of the 3M Company; Paul L. Parker, executive vice president of General Mills; Donnell Etzwiler; and Paul Batalden, then foundation president.

The development team's work paid off. In his 1983 president's report, Batalden noted that the McKnight grant had "made 1982 perhaps the most exciting and challenging yet for our twenty-three-year-old foundation."[112] Within six months $1.7 million of the additional $2.5 million needed had been raised, primarily from corporations headquartered in the Twin Cities. The medical center's employee fund-raising drive, chaired by Drs. Earl Young, Fred Rice, and Charles Converse, raised $117,000 by the end of 1983.[113]

Batalden credited James Toscano for much of the success of the capital campaign, saying, "As we made the rounds to the foundations and so on, it was a situation where it wasn't whether people would give us money, it was how much we needed. It was a wonderful situation to be in a thing that was that well staffed and that well supported."

North Tower Construction

Planning for the new building to house the International Diabetes Center (IDC) had barely gotten underway when it hit a major snag. Just as it had been when the Northland building was first envisioned in 1966, the old Beltline Pay

Dump was still percolating quietly under the proposed site. The Minnesota Pollution Control Agency determined that long-term site remediation would have to be undertaken to prevent hazardous compounds from moving into the local surface and groundwater. Just days before the official groundbreaking, plans for the new building were scrapped in favor of adding a five-story tower onto the existing Arneson Pavillion, which had been added on the north side of the Northland Building in 1978. Though relocated, the groundbreaking took place as scheduled on Columbus Day. Minnesota's Governor Rudy Perpich, renowned for his interest in developing international business for the state, attended the groundbreaking and declared October 12, 1983, "International Diabetes Center Day in Minnesota."[114]

By the end of 1983 estimated construction costs had risen to more than $13 million. Although this added to growing financial pressures at the medical center, the board continued to support the project. Board Member James Reinertsen spoke for the majority saying he "was willing to make a personal sacrifice to build the new building because it represented an investment in the future." Rodney Dueck, an ophthalmologist who was then secretary of the clinic board, called it a "wonderful opportunity for growth," pointing out that the community had already contributed more than $8 million to the project.[115] For James Toscano the mild frustration of trying to meet a fund-raising target that moved upwards almost as fast as the money came in was mitigated by the enthusiasm the project generated.

By the time the tower was dedicated in September 1985, it had grown to 111,983 square feet, including the 224-seat Naegele Auditorium and a spacious Dwan Conference Center, both on the seventh floor of the new "North Tower."[116] The total project cost had topped $15.5 million, about $10 million of which had been raised from the community. With the help and support of the medical center and the foundation, and through his own determination, Donnell Etzwiler's idea for improving the treatment of diabetes and other chronic diseases became a center of excellence with a growing international presence. The International Diabetes Center was now a reality. As Executive Director Toscano put it, "We purposefully grew the place very rapidly as an investment and it paid off."

Under the umbrella of the foundation, the IDC expanded and established an active research department. In 1979, the Eli Lilly Company selected the center as one of six research sites in the country to test its new biosynthetic insulin, a potentially life-saving drug. In 1981, the center was honored again when the National Institutes of Health selected it as one of twenty-one centers participating in a major ten-year study, the Diabetes Control and Complications Trial (DCCT), which tested the effect of aggressive blood glucose control on the long-term complications of diabetes. Results of the Diabetes Control and Complications Trial were published in 1993 and proved that the debilitating and life-threatening complications of diabetes can be prevented or delayed through aggressive management, giving new urgency to the center's mission of patient-centered care and education. Today under the leadership of endocrinologist Richard M. Bergenstal, the International Diabetes Center continues to carry its mission forward through integrated efforts in clinical care, education, research, and publishing.

PRIMARY DONORS TO THE NORTH TOWER CONSTRUCTION

McKnight Foundation
$5,000,000
Bush Foundation
$ 300,000
St. Louis Park Medical Center
$ 250,000
Medtronic, Inc.
$ 200,000
3M Company
$ 225,000
Carlson Companies
$ 200,000
Blandin Foundation
$ 150,000
Dwan Trust
$ 150,000
Jostens
$ 50,000
Naegele
$ 750,000

HEALTH PROMOTION AND PATIENT EDUCATION

The implementation of the HMO concept by St. Louis Park Medical Center and others in the early 1970s brought with it the implicit promise of a different kind of medical practice, one that involved the promotion of health. Partially at risk for the cost of its HMO members' injury and disease episodes, the medical center struggled to adapt traditional practice styles to the new reality. Expanding the

As a natural offshoot of their work in patient and professional education, the International Diabetes Center and the Health Education Center began developing and producing educational materials to support their respective programs. The diabetes center was the first to offer its materials for purchase to patients and health professionals. The books and booklets proved very popular and, in 1987, a local publisher was contracted to distribute the diabetes center's materials nationally. The market continued to expand. Today the IDC publishes patient education materials and consumer trade books under its imprint, IDC Publishing, reaching its market through several distributor contracts.

The Health Education Center began marketing its materials to businesses and health care organizations through a direct mail catalog in 1994. In 1995 IDC Publishing placed its products in the catalog in an effort to cooperatively expand the markets of both publishing programs. Today publishing marketing strategies include catalog and special offer mailings, attendance at national conferences, bookstore distribution, and the Internet.

definition of health care to include the services of health educators and other nonphysicians was the key to maintaining member health. Though this model was already in place in the diabetes center, it was not easy to implement it on a broader scale.

"It was an added expense," Glen Nelson said of the health education program that was started in 1974. "But it was an effort that was solidly based in the philosophy of the founders who asked, 'How do we practice better medicine?' not 'How can we be more profitable as a group?'" Throughout the 1970s the group, in cooperation with Medcenter Health Plan, developed a broad array of health promotion activities.

In 1973, Core Communications in Health, a Maryland company that had developed a one-on-one patient education model using audiovisual programming, proposed that St. Louis Park Medical Center serve as a program test site. This was approved and a new education center was set up in the then Diabetes Education Center under the medical direction of Donnell Etzwiler. Pat Herge (Angvik), a registered nurse, served as the group's first patient education coordinator. To support the program, Medcenter Health Plan agreed to set aside $20,000 for patient education costs above those absorbed by St. Louis Park Medical Center.[117]

St. Louis Park Medical Center purchased the Core Communications program in 1977, forming the nucleus of a new patient education department. Directed by registered nurse Mary Jane Madden, the department also assumed responsibility for managing several other programs in patient education and health promotion including a parenting group, a weight-loss program, and a hypertension clinic. In 1977 more than twenty organizations visited the new center, considering it a model and test site for innovative education strategies.[118]

As the center's medical director—a position created in 1975—one of A. Stuart Hanson's responsibilities was to direct the programs of the clinic. Encouraged by the effectiveness of the patient education department, Hanson began planning a new education department to include nutrition services, patient education, and in-service education for staff. This idea evolved over the next two years under the direction of Mary Jane Madden, Dr. Fritz Engstrom, and Marion Franz, a registered dietitian in the Diabetes Education Center. In 1980, a consolidated health education department was created by the medical center board, and it developed or absorbed many clinic programs. Examples include the newborn and family care program, which made a nurse clinician available to newborn infants and their families following early discharge from the hospital; the psoriasis and low-back-pain home care programs; and stress management programs. In addition, the surgery department began automatic referrals for presurgical education as a method to enhance informed consent and to accurately shape patient expectations.

"To this day, some practitioners are very comfortable having others do a lot of the teaching, and some physicians are not comfortable at all having anybody else involved. [But] it's been shown that if physicians don't use a team approach, they don't really do as well for the patients. They don't get the same sort of compliance and results. Some do, but on the whole, they don't."

A. Stuart Hanson, M.D.

Despite its growth and popularity with patients, the health education department continued to be a financial drain on the clinic. In recognition of this, the medical center board transferred the department to the foundation in 1984, where it was renamed "Health Education Center." The foundation, with its education mission and nonprofit status, made it possible to attract outside grants to support expansion of health education experiments while keeping the existing programs accessible to both the medical center and the health plan. As hoped, foundation sponsorship enabled the Health Education Center, now under the leadership of Paul Terry, Ph.D., to grow rapidly and improve its financial performance.

SHAPE: Promoting Executive Health

The health and fitness culture of the late 1970s developed in parallel to the health education movement at the medical center. Medical Center President Glen Nelson was an

"Patient education is good medicine and good economics. Our basic philosophy is that patient knowledge and participation promote better outcomes. Patient compliance, understanding, and knowledge are fundamental."[119]

Glen Nelson, M.D., Minnesota Medicine, *1986*

active marathon runner and a promoter of exercise and fitness training as a significant factor in attaining and maintaining health. So it was to a receptive audience that Mary Jane Madden and A. Stuart Hanson presented their proposal for a new executive health program in late 1978.

Inspired by a program developed by the Sun Valley Executive Health Institute, Madden and Hanson proposed that a series of healthy lifestyle training programs be organized and marketed to area companies that had traditionally turned to St. Louis Park Medical Center for executive physicals and other special health benefits. Information gathered during the initial phase of the program would be used to develop a multimedia program for employees at all levels.[120]

The initial training sessions were held at Minnesuing, the Carlson Companies retreat center in northern Wisconsin, in the early spring of 1979. Half of the spaces were reserved for St. Louis Park Medical Center physicians, on the theory that exposure to the training would reduce their natural resistance to prevention and health care services based on behavior modification. Skeptics, in particular, were encouraged to go. One of these skeptics was James Reinertsen, a rheumatologist and an avid athlete who had been with the medical center less than a year.

By April 1979 Reinertsen was heading a committee proposing medical center support for the program. Reinertsen cited the growing numbers of providers, consumers, educators, and corporate leaders who were showing an interest in comprehensive health improvement, and he pushed his agenda forward. "This was a fairly dangerous adventure in the sense . . . [that] there wasn't a wide base of support for it," Reinertsen recalled. "So Stu [Hanson] said . . . 'I'll give it to the new guy. He doesn't have any enemies yet. So if it goes down, it won't go down because they hate him for something else he's done; it will go down because it was a bad idea.'" The early response to the program from the physicians and the executives who participated was positive enough to convince the medical center board to approve developing the idea further.

Later that year the program was named SHAPE—shorthand for Self Help and Physical Evaluation—and organized as a for-profit business. SHAPE was a combined effort of the medical center, Medcenter Health Plan, and Methodist Hospital. Larry Vorlicky, medical director of the health plan who had been involved from the beginning, convinced his board to contribute $25,000 to the project. Methodist Hospital put up $50,000 in working capital. Another $25,000 from St. Louis Park Medical Center brought the total capitalization to $100,000. Reinertsen, as SHAPE's president and medical director, began signing clients up for the new worksite health promotion program, including Dayton's, Medtronic, Valspar, and Sperry Univac.

It was tough going in the early years. The SHAPE program was designed as an intensive learning and experiential course in nutrition, exercise, and stress management for executives. As a result the package was elaborate and expensive and proved to be of little interest to a broader market. "We tried to go at the market by introducing it to the senior leadership and then say 'Gee, wouldn't it be nice if we could take pieces of this and implement it in your work environment?'" Vorlicky stated several years later. But the financial benefits of health improvement programs were not very well appreciated at the time.

Despite the obstacles, SHAPE continued to make progress over the next few years. Under its first executive director, Dan Halvorson, SHAPE created a program for the general workplace and offered it to Methodist Hospital and St. Louis Park Medical Center employees in the fall of 1980. Within a year, ninety-one employees had participated in the program and received a complete health assessment and health profile. SHAPE began carefully franchising its programs and services in 1981, and clinics in California, Missouri, and North Dakota responded.[121] Over the next few years the SHAPE staff created the program Reinertsen had envisioned in 1979, "a comprehensive, high-quality, scientifically proven health improvement program for the general community."[122] One early client, the Scott and White Clinic of Temple, Texas, wrote, "We sought a program balanced with equal emphasis on good nutrition, stress management, and freedom from imprudent use of stimulants and depressants. SHAPE is just what we wanted."[123] Affiliates in 1984 included the Mason Clinic in Seattle, the Fargo Clinic in North Dakota, and the Geisinger Medical Center in Danville, Pennsylvania.

Financial success was slower to arrive. SHAPE continued to require support from the medical center whose total investment grew to $75,000 by 1983.[124] In 1984 the now-merged health plan, MedCenters, reevaluated its commitment to the SHAPE project and voted to cut its losses, turning its share of the program content and the SHAPE name over to the medical center. "We learned in the first year or two that it was very difficult to run a company that had three different owners who had different purposes for starting the company," Reinertsen said, looking back at the program's progress. "SHAPE was losing money, and nobody wanted to participate in the losses."

In 1985 SHAPE became a division of the fast-growing foundation. Over the years its finances reversed and new clients and programs were added. In 1994 SHAPE was renamed Park Nicollet *HealthSource*, which continues to offer worksite health promotion programs and health-testing services along with educational materials to its local and national customers.

11

LIVING A PHILOSOPHY

"NOT-QUITE PRIVATE PRACTICE"

ROOTED IN THE CULTURE OF ST. LOUIS PARK MEDICAL Center was a steadfast commitment to training, education, and research—what James Reinertsen would later describe as "not-quite private practice." From the beginning an academic component was woven into almost every facet of practice. Staff meetings often began with the presentation of an interesting case or a research paper. New members of the professional staff were asked to identify an area of academic interest and to choose a research topic, and they were expected to pursue an academic appointment at the University of Minnesota, the Veterans Administration Hospital, or Minneapolis General. In return, the organization offered paid time away from the office and a work environment that included some of the collegial aspects of a university faculty within a private practice group.

For many the desire to learn, teach, and grow as professionals occupied leisure as well as work hours. According to Robert (Bud) Green, "We didn't play golf on our afternoons off. Most of us when we had an afternoon off would go to the university, do something in the lab here, or work over one of the clinical research projects going on."

As a consequence of this early emphasis on academic time and professional education, each physician became an accomplished subspecialist, often among the first in the metro area to receive certification as new subspecialty certification boards were created. However, the opportunity to develop a full-time subspecialty practice depended on referrals. Throughout the 1950s and 1960s, the group experimented with different strategies for increasing referrals—including offering themselves as speakers to general practitioners in outlying towns where there was less fear of losing patients to the growing medical center. By 1955 sixty physicians in the region were actively sending patients to the group. Several departments developed their regional contacts into regular rounds, seeing patients and consulting with referring physicians in communities such as Hutchinson and Thief River Falls. These outreach activities were very much appreciated by the communities served.

CLINICAL CONFERENCE SERIES

The coincidental births of the clinical conference and the St. Louis Park Medical Center *Bulletin* were, in part, an extension of the group's outreach activities. Chief of Staff Frank Johnson came up with the idea of a quarterly bulletin in 1956 and was enthusiastically supported by Robert Green. The first St. Louis Park Medical Center clinical conference, the brainchild of Alvin Schultz, took place at Mt. Sinai Hospital in the fall of 1956 and presented the perfect opportunity for establishing the publication. The conference proceedings were designated Volume One, Number One, of the St. Louis Park Medical Center *Bulletin* and mailed to over 1,200 physicians in Minnesota and the region.

Following their initial success, Schultz and conference co-chair Wyman Jacobson put together a series of monthly conferences covering subjects of interest to the general practitioner. Clinic physicians presented topics such as "The Management of Peptic Ulcers," "Maternal Mortality," and "Chemotherapy of Leukemia" throughout

1957. The conferences were not particularly well attended, but the papers presented were circulated widely and provided the basis for several issues of the new *Bulletin*, which was edited by Alvin Schultz until he left the partnership in 1959. The group became known to physicians in rural areas in large part through the *Bulletin*, according to Administrator Roger Asplin. As confidence in the group grew, so did the number of referrals.

"Medical education is a crucial function of the St. Louis Park Medical Center, supported by tradition, recognized in the original statement of objectives . . . essential to the recruitment of able new personnel and retention of present personnel, mandatory to prevent physician obsolescence, necessary for accreditation and basic to the lives of physicians."

William Fifer, M.D.

While the *Bulletin* is still published today, the clinical conferences at Mount Sinai ended when the majority of St. Louis Park Medical Center physicians moved their hospital loyalties to Methodist in 1960. In 1963 surgeon Robert Benjamin spearheaded a new conference series—the Wednesday Noon Clinical Conferences—which were held over lunch in the Arneson Library. Many of the meetings started with the group's viewing unidentified slides from a specific case. Each physician present would submit a diagnosis, and a discussion would follow. A prepared talk would sometimes be given on an interesting case. Each death of a clinic patient would be examined.

The larger departments also organized regular conferences, or "grand rounds." Norman Sterrie, for instance, organized weekly pediatrics grand rounds at Methodist Hospital in 1963. The surgery department met every Friday to discuss all unusual cases, deaths, and complications. The internal medicine department held medical rounds at Methodist twice a month and a weekly journal club, which the other specialties were encouraged to attend. "The importance of such meetings," John LaBree wrote in 1964, "cannot be overstressed."[125]

SEEKING SUBSPECIALIZATION

The ability to provide opportunities for the development of individual subspecialty interests was at the heart of group practice. Practically every physician took some advantage of this support, often bringing new and valuable skills back to the group. Thoracic surgeon Jerry Grismer spent nine months in 1962 and 1963 studying valvular surgery with C. Walton Lillehi of the University of Minnesota just a few years after Lillehi's team had introduced the technique of open-heart surgery to the world. Two years later thoracic surgeon Earl Young left for six months to study vascular surgery at Baylor University with renowned heart surgeon Michael DeBakey. On his return Young was the first physician in the metropolitan area to begin using the new techniques developed at Baylor.[126] In 1964 pediatrician Richard Cushing left for a residency in pediatric allergy at the University of Michigan.

Salary and benefits often continued during all or part of the time spent away from the clinic for subspecialty training. In 1966 Robert Benjamin asked for a sabbatical leave to study as a surgical fellow at the Roswell Park Hospital in Buffalo, New York. The St. Louis Park Medical Center Board approved the request and agreed to provide 75 percent of his base salary for the two-month program. When James Dahl requested a two-month leave to implement techniques in coronary care at the University of Minnesota Cardiology Department, the board approved a leave of up to three months at full salary.[127]

Even as the group matured and became committed to offering comprehensive care to members of the Medcenter Health Plan, St. Louis Park Medical Center retained its self-perception as a clinic of specialists and subspecialists. Indeed, by some accounts, one of the attractions of the health maintenance organization was the opportunity to rapidly expand the group's patient base to a point where even the most obscure subspecialty might be added. Although this internal focus on the development of subspecialists created a shortage of physicians in primary care departments and a high-cost structure in the 1980s, the emphasis on bringing in and developing academically-oriented specialists held. By 1993 the group included forty-five specialties in their roster of services.

ESTABLISHING RESIDENCIES

The fall of 1963 marked the beginning of the first surgical residency program at St. Louis Park Medical Center. Earl Young, who had developed the program and organized its tentative acceptance by both the American Board of Surgeons and the American College of Surgeons, was named preceptor of surgical resident training. The medical center provided an $800-per-month stipend to residents who rotated through surgical departments over a one-year period.

In July 1967 the program, offered in cooperation with Methodist Hospital, became affiliated with the University of Minnesota. Wyman Jacobson called it "one of the most significant milestones in the growth of our organization." The university affiliation was "a tribute to the entire staff, a distinct honor and one of the most respected expressions of confidence from the professional leaders in medicine and surgery."[128] Roger Asplin remembers that "Earl Young was quite close to Dr. [John] Najarian . . . those two established the surgical residencies we had here." Young, who continued as preceptor, viewed the program as "a commitment to the highest standards of education and training by the members of the St. Louis Park Medical Center."[129]

The surgical residency program "was a feather in our cap," according to Robert Benjamin. "For quite a while there we were the only people outside of the university who were allowed to train their residents. Just think of the advantage that gave us. . . . We'd see how they worked and we could pick the best ones." The program later became the model for residency programs organized by the obstetrics and gynecology and family practice departments.

INDIVIDUAL TEACHING

The commitment of the group to teaching medicine extended beyond the clinic's established residency programs. Most physicians had teaching appointments at the University of Minnesota. In 1967, for example, the internal medicine department listed eight clinical instructors, one clinical assistant professor, three clinical associate professors, and two full clinical professors reporting for duty at the university. William Fifer, for one, succeeded J. A. Meyers as director of the Chest Clinic at the university in 1957 and the next year provided three chapters on lung disease for the revised edition of Cecil Watson's *Outlines of Internal Medicine.*[130] Alex Barno and Don Freeman lectured in obstetrics for general practitioners at the university's Continuation Center, and Arnold Anderson taught in the circuit teaching program at the invitation of the Wisconsin State Medical Society.

The teaching pursuits of St. Louis Park Medical Center physicians were not limited to Minnesota and the surrounding region. Orthopedic surgeon Walter Indeck was invited by the University of Copenhagen to become a Fulbright professor in 1965. The professorship involved a nine-month stay in Denmark to organize a training program in orthopedic surgery for residents at the Orthopedic Hospital there.[131] Dr. Ramon Gustillo, who joined the group in 1964, was in demand in his native Philippines, returning there on several occasions to teach orthopedic surgery.

The group showed as much enthusiasm for the professional education of other health professionals as they did for physicians. Several educational programs aimed at improving the many facets of health care were established and supported by the medical center.

Orthopedic Assistants

Rising sports injury rates and an explosion of new procedures in the late 1960s dramatically increased the workload in the orthopedic department. To make the best use of the physician's time, the department wanted to train orthopedic assistants to handle routine patient care and to assist in surgery. George Reisdorf, orthopedic surgeon; Loren Vorlicky, chair of the Research and Development Committee; and Nat Wisser, a member of the foundation board, organized a training program in cooperation with Normandale Junior College in Bloomington. The program was funded primarily by the State of Minnesota. It received continuing support from the foundation beginning in 1970.

In 1961, Norman Sterrie became the first St. Louis Park Medical Center physician to achieve subspecialty certification. Although his subspecialty practice—pediatric allergies—quickly became a major asset to the clinic, Sterrie recalled it as a mixed blessing for him personally: "One of the most difficult things for me was watching my general pediatrics practice disappear, with allergy taking over in time." Arnold Anderson underscored this holistic view: "We pioneered the subspecialization of pediatrics, but we felt it was important for a pediatrician to be a general pediatrician half the time and a subspecialist the other half, in order to bring a perspective of general child care and growth and development to our subspecialty."

Orthoptics Training Program

Orthoptic technician Dwayne Broe joined the teaching staff of the St. Paul-Ramsey Squint Clinic in 1965 where he taught techniques of orthoptic therapies and contact lens fitting to University of Minnesota ophthalmology residents. Four years later the program expanded to include a once-a-week rotation of ophthalmology residents to the St. Louis Park Medical Center orthoptic offices to work under Broe's guidance.

Pharmacy Program

The group's pharmacy also became a training facility for the University of Minnesota. In 1969 the School of Pharmacy set up a rotation with Medcenter Pharmacy for twenty-five senior students to study clinical pharmacy with Raymond Anderson. Anderson increased his personal commitment to professional education in 1971, accepting a one-afternoon-per-week teaching position in the university's pharmacy program.

NONPHYSICIAN STAFF EDUCATION

The delivery of medical care in a group clinic necessarily involves a team effort, and the training and professional education of nonphysician staff were not neglected. Informal seminars for nurses and other interested team members were conducted on an as-needed basis within each department, and other more formal programs were implemented.

Sandwich Seminars

In his new capacity as director of medical education in 1969, William Fifer organized a program of weekly "sandwich seminars," held every Thursday for nurses and other interested people. At each of these meetings one of the specialists would present a topic in his specialty, followed by a discussion. Fifer also organized a weekly training program for medical receptionists. "The receptionist," Fifer wrote, "is the real determiner of which patient sees which doctor and how soon. This crucial job demands more medical education."[132]

Business Administration

The business administration office during this period implemented a range of on-going education programs for employees including new-employee orientation, programs to teach "management by objectives" to supervisors, and training programs in medical terminology and secretarial skills in cooperation with North Hennepin Vocational School. Roger Asplin also developed a relationship with the University of Minnesota's master's degree program in health administration, creating a hands-on clinic management residency program at St. Louis Park Medical Center beginning in 1973. Active in professional organizations, Asplin was elected president of the Medical Group Managers Association in 1978. In 1977, James Stolhanske, then assistant administrator at St. Louis Park Medical Center, contributed a chapter on personnel management in the text *Medical Group Practice Management.*[133]

RESPONSIBLE SELF-EVALUATION

"Life is short, and the art is long; the occasion fleeting; experience fallacious; and judgment difficult. The physician must not only be prepared to do what is right himself but also to make patients, the attendants, and the externals cooperate."

Hippocrates

Since its inception, St. Louis Park Medical Center had been self-consciously organizing itself to do—in the words of Hippocrates—"what is right." A group practice based on academic achievement, life-long involvement in education and research, and cooperation across disciplines would by definition, the group thought, yield quality medicine. In the less-complicated era of the 1950s and 1960s, quality was assured by the open and intellectual atmosphere maintained in a small, multidisciplinary group. Quality, according to founder John LaBree, was assured "by sharing everything we did and seeing patients together constantly." But there were also sporadic efforts to examine the practice itself. In 1958, founder Alex Barno initiated a study of record-room procedures. The study identified eleven specific problems, quantified the extent of each problem, and offered a recommended solution based on interviews with the support staff and physicians.[134]

Physical therapy, directed by Roger Ambrosan, was the first department to evaluate its work and make a report to the board. The 1959 report, which Arnold Anderson suggested "should serve as a model for all of us," included the types of cases treated, methods of treatment, numbers treated, and outcomes.[135] Throughout his term as president, Anderson advocated the development of a "standard or critical yardstick more or less applicable to all," a vision still well ahead of the state of the art and the resources of the group.[136]

As the group grew larger, they began to notice the divergence between their methods of quality assurance, actual outcomes, and the patient's perception of service delivered. "Our bigness works against us in trying to create a homey, friendly, and sympathetic atmosphere," Robert Benjamin wrote in the in-house newsletter *Clini Call* in 1962. "It is far more difficult, and impossible in most cases, for patients to

"Medicine isn't cold and white when there's a calm telephone voice to help a frantic mother; when there's a laboratory worker able to convince a small child that she's not about to take a drop more blood than she needs to help him; when an elderly patient is met at the door with a wheelchair and efficiently scheduled for tiring tests; when a doctor senses and relieves needless worries that a patient finds hard to put into words.... Medicine isn't cold and white—but the warmth and brightness aren't chiefly from the decor. They're from you."[138]

J. Roger Asplin, Clini Call, *1967*

determine whether or not they are receiving 'good medical care.' Given this difficulty, it is not surprising that they evaluate their care by the subjective feelings they have toward the people who take care of them."[137]

While patient satisfaction was the designated responsibility of every staff member, it fell to the physician-managers to organize systems of care that could be "measured against carefully established objective standards."[139] William Fifer urged the group to allow him to begin the development of a scientific quality assurance program in 1969. The board, feeling impoverished by the construction of the Northland Building, was unable to financially support his plans, and Fifer left later that year to pursue his interest in quality assurance at the Northlands Regional Medical Program.

A few weeks after joining the group in 1971, A. Stuart Hanson was urged by Bud Green, in his role as chair of the Medical Staff Committee, to apply for funds that were then available for the study of the medical audit as it applied to outpatient care. With co-investigator and fellow internist Edward Kraus, Hanson spent the next two years of his academic time directing a $50,000 study to create a meaningful system of performance evaluation based on the traditional retrospective medical audit.

"We tried to develop a system which would give us some idea how the aggregate did, but also how the individual physicians did with numbers of cases," Hanson explained. "So we reviewed the literature and developed a methodology of surveying the [medical] records, but we didn't think the results were any good. We published [the results] and the group looked at it and said this is a waste of time, and we said, 'You're right, we agree.'" The consensus at the time was that it would be more effective to simply ask the staff and patients what the problems were. The retrospective audit techniques Hanson and his team had developed could then be targeted more specifically and cost effectively in support of solving acknowledged problems. At that point, according to Hanson, "We were a clinic that was primed for the next iteration."

"The Quality Assurance Program doesn't cost us dollars, it saves us dollars. It costs less to do things right, and that is what the Quality Assurance Program does for us. . . . it helps us do things right."[141]

Glen Nelson, M.D.

QUALITY ASSURANCE PROGRAM

By 1975 the need for a comprehensive approach to quality assurance was urgent. Quality assurance programs were required by the American Group Practice Association, state regulations for HMOs, and peer review organizations.[140] The development of the health plan had put the group at financial risk for the quality of care they provided and, after many years of little or no activity, the group's Professional Liability Committee was suddenly faced with ten lawsuits in 1975.

In 1974, William Fifer and Loren Vorlicky recruited Dr. Paul Batalden, who had directed a study of quality assurance programs at the Department of Health, Education and Welfare in Washington, D.C., to come to Minneapolis and test his theories of quality assurance in a clinical setting. In 1975 Batalden submitted and won a $306,000 grant from the W. K. Kellogg Foundation to establish the St. Louis Park Medical Center Quality Assurance Program. The program was designed to develop what Batalden thought was the missing ingredient in quality assessment—a mechanism for changing behavior. "Assessment alone," he said in 1980, "is of little value to quality assurance unless it leads to changes that improve patient care."[142]

The first step in the quality assurance process was to develop and test methods for identifying and remedying medical care delivery problems. The quality assurance staff gathered information from the support staff, from physicians, and from patients and presented it to a departmental meeting. Participants were then able to identify the problems that most interfered with the delivery of care. Although such meetings are now commonplace, at the time some of the departments at St. Louis Park Medical Center had never met as a group. "The doctors met," Batalden recounted, "but when you were starting to work on the systems of care for patients and the way patients experienced the place, [the doctors] had no view of the way things actually worked, so you couldn't begin to work on standards of care until you had some kind of context or environment that was really functional. So the question 'What do we all agree needs to be improved?' really helped launch a cooperative effort."

Medical record problems were identified so often that the quality assurance staff suggested a comprehensive review of the existing record. As described by nurse Carol Hersman, the new record, implemented in 1978, used a "shingled-half-sheet" format that allowed a patient's last ten visits to the clinic to be visible at a glance. After one year, 77 percent of the physician staff strongly agreed that the new record was an "improved working tool in my practice." There was also "limited but important evidence," as Batalden cautiously reported to the Kellogg Foundation in 1979, that the Quality Assurance Program had succeeded in "improving the significance of internal professional meetings and seminars."[143]

As part of the effort to find potential health-care delivery problems, the quality assurance staff developed and tested a series of patient interview formats. Work done by William Fifer in 1976 for the National Center for Health Research had demonstrated that "communication blocks have a significant effect on the quality of health care."[144] The Quality Assurance Program was interested in determining "how often these blocks occur, how serious they are, and what can be done to overcome them."[145] Over the course of three years, more than 1,100 patient interviews were conducted, identifying 1,900 problems of which approximately 30 percent were related to access, 17 percent to services provided, 18 percent to discrepancies between what the chart said and what the patient remembered, and

11 percent to patient compliance. The results, published in 1980 in the *Journal of Community Health*, were used extensively to guide the quality assurance work at St. Louis Park Medical Center.

Health Services Research Center

In February 1976 Hanson asked the medical center Board to make a financial commitment to create a research center, which would include the Quality Assurance Program. This was approved and the Health Services Research Center became part of the foundation in August 1976. Batalden, now a part-time employee of the foundation, set about organizing the next phase in quality assurance research.

With the help of a second grant of $665,000 from the W. K. Kellogg Foundation, the Health Services Research Center began a national program, designed to transfer the medical center's experience in quality assurance to other group practice clinics. The Quality Assurance Program Development Project selected ten clinics in various parts of the country and assisted them in establishing and implementing their own quality assurance programs based on the St. Louis Park Medical Center model. The medical center leadership—including Glen Nelson, Loren Vorlicky, Roger Asplin, and A. Stuart Hanson—participated in site-orientation meetings to reinforce the fundamental principle that leadership commitment is critical to the success of a quality assurance program. For each site the Health Services Research Center staff prepared a customized workshop to develop the site's resources and data sources, as well as the commitment of the group to the project. Continuing consultation services were provided throughout the project.

The comments of participants are perhaps the best indication of the project's success. The Straub Clinic noted that the project had set up a "formal mechanism for communication between nursing and physician staff as well as adminis-

"We wanted to focus on the outcome from the patient's perspective. . . . What had been traditional in health-care quality activities up until that time was for the doctors to come to an agreement about what would constitute a standard and then go measure whether the care complied with that or not. And that really didn't yield a heck of a lot that was fresh or exciting, and usually just got a lot of push-back resistance and finger-pointing. . . . Listening to patients' comments about their care was the forerunner basically of much of the current patient satisfaction interest that's going on in the country now."

Paul Batalden, M.D.

QUALITY ASSURANCE PROGRAM DEVELOPMENT PROJECT

Jackson Clinic,
Madison, Wisconsin
Marshfield Clinic,
Marshfield, Wisconsin
Straub Clinic and Hospital,
Honolulu, Hawaii
Chickasha Clinic,
Chickasha, Oklahoma
Salt Lake Clinic,
Salt Lake City, Utah
Rockridge Health Care Plan,
Oakland, California
Community Health Plan of South Dade,
Miami, Florida
Family Health Center,
Kalamazoo, Michigan
Field Medical Group,
Chicago, Illinois
Lovelace Medical Foundation,
Albuquerque, New Mexico[146]

tration," and had afforded participants "a view of their department and how it functions in the entire organization which we do not think heretofore existed." It voted to continue the program on its own in 1981. The Lovelace Medical Center reported that the program had "been well accepted by the medical staff, administration, and middle management," and it, too, voted to continue the quality assurance program in 1982. The fast-growing Marshfield Clinic voted unanimously in 1982 to continue, as did the Salt Lake, Chickasha, and Jackson clinics. With this model, Marshfield observed in the project's final report, "People know there is an on-going mechanism to address concerns. This is as important as the solutions themselves."[147]

The experience generated by the Health Services Research Center in quality assurance was presented to a national audience in 1981. Seminars were held in Minneapolis, Arlington (Virginia), San Antonio, and San Diego, and included a faculty drawn from the leadership of each of the ten participating clinics. For the next several years the Health Services Research Center continued to work informally with this group, meeting once each year to exchange ideas, successes, and failures.[148]

Quality Assurance Milestones

Quality assurance research at St. Louis Park Medical Center did not diminish with the advent of the national program. In 1978 the Health Services Research Center initiated a drug utilization review study to create a prescribing profile for each physician in a subspecialty department. The data was gathered over a three-month period and analyzed by the Quality Assurance Program's advisory board. The advisory board worked closely with the medical center's Primary Care Committee to develop guidelines for periodic health care evaluations, chronic medication refills, physical therapy referrals, and patient self-care materials.

In his annual report to the board of the St. Louis Park Medical Center Research Foundation in 1982, Batalden cited several successful new programs generated by the Quality Assurance Program such as the psoriasis home care program, a series of patient information brochures for minor surgeries, and a day-of-admission system for surgery. The "Art of Caring" interview programs were also developed in 1982, offering St. Louis Park Medical Center physicians important customer feedback.[149] The technique continues today to be a valuable learning tool.

"First there is a kind of early denial that your quality isn't good, then there's a recognition phase during which there's a lot of lip service paid to what you are going to do about it. Here you have a group of people who are used to making anecdotal decisions and doing things the way they want and not being evaluated, so you would expect that there might be some clash. Batalden brought an advanced way of looking at what we are now talking about in terms of outcomes and in the process made a meaningful contribution in the evolution of the whole organization."

Glen Nelson, M.D.

"NOT-QUITE PRIVATE PRACTICE"

St. Louis Park Medical Center had much to be proud of on the occasion of its thirtieth anniversary, and the celebration was appropriately grand. On June 26, 1981, the medical center family gathered at Orchestra Hall in Minneapolis to share stories, sing along with Mitch Miller, and dance to the sounds of the Minnesota Orchestra. By 1981 the group had grown to 135 physicians, 32 allied health professionals, and 750 employees. The founders of the group took a bow, everyone enjoyed champagne and birthday cake, and the dancing went on until midnight.

With its combination of private group practice, clinical teaching, and research, St. Louis Park Medical Center was recognized nationally as a "premier multispecialty group."[150] The center's growing reputation was a source of great satisfaction to the founders and attracted young, academically inclined physicians to its employ. Founder Robert Green reported in 1980 that "some of the best-qualified physicians available anywhere [were] making the decision to come here." [151]

During a discussion of the medical center's mission in 1982, James Reinertsen coined the descriptive phrase "not-quite private practice" to communicate the group's long and passionately held tradition of collegial participation in training, education, and research alongside the daily practice of medicine. Although he had not yet heard the words, A. Stuart Hanson summed up the concept of a not-quite private practice at the annual meeting in 1980:

> As the medical center evolves and grows, not only in numbers but in expertise, we need to look back and continually remind ourselves what are the important tenets. . . . We have reaffirmed that clinical practice is essential. . . .We have reaffirmed that our organization adheres to a high standard of excellence in conducting our medical practices. If anything, this is our highest priority. We have reaffirmed that a scientific basis of making our health care decisions and the access and dissemination of the knowledge needed to conduct a humane medical practice is valued highly. We have reaffirmed that medical education does not end with medical school or residency training, but is a continuing requirement of a quality health care professional. We have continued our dedication to evaluate and assess what we are doing . . . and to improve what we do from all quarters of our organization. . . . We do not always reach our desired goals and what we value in our professional organization is not always achieved in reality. But it is important not to lose sight of the commitments this organization has made and to reaffirm and expand on those ideals as we move on to another year in a decade that will be very significant.[152]

Chapter 6

1 "Lilac Way Shopping Center to Be Expanded," *Minneapolis Star*, November 12, 1949. "Architects Completing Plans for a New $100,000 Addition to the Lilac Way Shopping Center," *St. Louis Park Dispatch*, November 4, 1949.

2 Robert Green, "The Birth of the Medical Center," *Med-a-Cen*, February 15, 1961, 2.

3 "One Out of Three Park Residents Under 21," *St. Louis Park Dispatch*, October 21, 1949.

4 J. Roger Asplin, "A Brief History of St. Louis Park Medical Center," (Internal document October 7, 1975), 5.

5 Robert Green, interview with author, December 14, 1993.

6 Letter from Morten Arneson to Arnold Anderson, undated.

7 Ibid.

8 "Young Physicians Honor Couple for Faith, Confidence, Support," *Suburban Life*, June 17, 1962, sec. 3, 12.

9 Wollan and Wollan Company, "15th Anniversary History of the St. Louis Park Medical Center" (Preliminary draft, May 10, 1966).

10 Robert Green, "Birth of the Center," *Clini Call*, July 15, 1961, 2.

11 President's Commission on the Health Needs of the Nation, "Building America's Health" (Raleigh, North Carolina: Health Publications Institute, 1953), 14.

12 Wyman Jacobson, Chief of Staff's Report, St. Louis Park Medical Center, June 19, 1952.

13 The partnership was the only organizational structure acceptable to the group's lender because each of the partners could then be held individually liable for the entire debt. A Mayo-like corporate structure would have to wait until the partnership equity was sufficient to serve as collateral for additional debt.

14 George Halsey Hunt and Marcus Goldstein, *Medical Group Practice in the United States*, pub. no. 77 (Washington, D.C.: Federal Security Agency, Public Health Service, 1951), 9.

15 J. Roger Asplin, "A Brief History of St. Louis Park Medical Center," 5.

16 Robert Green, "St. Louis Park Medical Center: Twenty-Five Years of Service to the Community," *Minnesota Medicine* 60(May 1977): 351.

17 "125 Years of Service: A History of the Hennepin County Medical Society," *Bulletin of the Hennepin County Medical Society* 51(June 1980 anniversary supplement): 19.

18 Minutes of the Hennepin County Medical Society Board, May 26, 1955, 312.

19 Minutes of the St. Louis Park Medical Center Board, June 1, 1955.

20 Arnold Anderson, interview with author, February 11, 1994.

21 "Looking Back to the Days of 'Auld Lang Syne,'" *Clini Call*, January, 1979, 1.
22 Alex Barno, "The St. Louis Park Medical Center and Dr. D. W. Freeman" (Address to group at Dr. Freeman's Farewell Party, July 23, 1966).
23 Rosemary Stevens, *In Sickness and In Wealth: American Hospitals in the Twentieth Century* (New York: Basic Books, 1989), 227.
24 Barno, "The St. Louis Park Medical Center."
25 Ibid.

Chapter 7
26 George Lund as cited in Mark Peacock (Preliminary draft history of Park Nicollet, Park Nicollet Medical Foundation, 1989), 222.
27 Donald Freeman, interview with author, April 27, 1994.
28 John LaBree, Chief of Staff's Report, St. Louis Park Medical Center, May 20, 1954.
29 Richard Webber, Chief of Staff's Report, St. Louis Park Medical Center, May 21, 1953.
30 Richard Anderson, Financial Report, St. Louis Park Medical Center, April 18, 1957.
31 Richard Webber, Minutes of the St. Louis Park Medical Center Board, December 18, 1952.
32 Minutes of the St. Louis Park Medical Center Board, July 14, 1954.
33 Robert Green, personal communication with author, March 18, 1994.
34 *The Scope*, July 2, 1953, 1.
35 Richard Webber, Chief of Staff's Report, St. Louis Park Medical Center, May 21, 1953.
36 Memorandum from Frank Johnson to Executive Committee, St. Louis Park Medical Center, September 9, 1955.
37 Minutes of the St. Louis Park Medical Center Board, February 15, 1956.
38 Letter of resignation from Frank Johnson to the St. Louis Park Medical Center Board, September 12, 1956.
39 Arnold Anderson, interview with author, February 11, 1994.
40 Minutes of the St. Louis Park Medical Center Board, April 16, 1953.
41 Minutes of the St. Louis Park Medical Center Board, February 29, 1956.
42 Minutes of the St. Louis Park Medical Center Board, May 2, 1956.
43 Minutes of the St. Louis Park Medical Center Board, February 22, 1956.
44 *The Park: A History of the City of St. Louis Park* (Published by the City of St. Louis Park and Minneapolis, 1976), 43.

45 Robert Green, "Letter to Editor," *St. Louis Park Dispatch*, September 9, 1954.
46 Richard Anderson, Report to the Staff, Minutes of St. Louis Park Medical Center, April 18, 1958.
47 Arnold Anderson, Remarks to the Group Accepting Chief of Staff Position, Minutes of the St. Louis Park Medical Center Board, December 1957.
48 Ibid.
49 Ibid.
50 Arnold Anderson, Executive Committee Report on Business Administration, Minutes of the St. Louis Park Medical Center Board, May 15, 1958.
51 Minutes of the St. Louis Park Medical Center Board, October 16, 1958, and October 30, 1958.
52 Arnold Anderson, Remarks to the Group Accepting Chief of Staff Position, December 1957.
53 Robert Green, "Birth of the Center," *Clini Call*, July 15, 1961, 4.

Chapter 8
54 Annual Report of St. Louis Park Medical Center, 1965.
55 Arnold Anderson, Minutes of the St. Louis Park Medical Center Board, May 11, 1964.
56 J. Roger Asplin, interview with author, December 27, 1993.
57 Letter from Morten Arneson to Alex Barno, January 16, 1982.
58 Memorandum from Wyman Jacobson to Richard Webber, June 16, 1966.
59 J. Roger Asplin, Administrator's Annual Report, St. Louis Park Medical Center, 1968.
60 *Clini Call*, December, 1969.
61 J. Roger Asplin, Administrator's Annual Report, St. Louis Park Medical Center, 1969.
62 Wyman Jacobson, President's Annual Report, St. Louis Park Medical Center, February 17, 1966.
63 Wyman Jacobson, Annual Report of St. Louis Park Medical Center, 1966.
64 Alex Barno, "The St. Louis Park Medical Center and Dr. D. W. Freeman," (Address to group at Dr. Freeman's Farewell Party, July 23, 1966).
65 Arnold Anderson, Annual Report of St. Louis Park Medical Center, 1962.
66 J. Roger Asplin, Administrator's Annual Report, St. Louis Park Medical Center, 1969.
67 J. Roger Asplin, Administrator's Annual Report, St. Louis Park Medical Center, 1963.

68 J. Roger Asplin, Administrator's Annual Report, St. Louis Park Medical Center, 1971.
69 David L. vonWeiss, "Does Family Practice Work in a Multispecialty Clinic?" *Minnesota Medicine* 60(May 1977): 344.
70 Clifford Simack, "Help Comes with a Personal Touch for Patients at the St. Louis Park Clinic," *Minneapolis Tribune*, December 10, 1971.
71 James Dahl, Annual Report of St. Louis Park Medical Center, 1969.
72 Jerome Grismer, Annual Report of St. Louis Park Medical Center, 1965.
73 Norman Sterrie, President's Annual Report, St. Louis Park Medical Center, 1972.
74 Leonard Benedict, Laboratory Annual Report, St. Louis Park Medical Center, 1962.
75 Leonard Benedict, Laboratory Annual Report, St. Louis Park Medical Center, 1969.
76 Leonard Benedict, "Some Functions of Our Clinical Laboratory," *Clini Call*, February 28, 1964, 2.
77 Robert Benjamin, Minutes of the St. Louis Park Medical Center Board, March 9, 1959.
78 *Clini Call*, April 22, 1960, 3.
79 Loren Vorlicky, interview with author, October 5, 1994.
80 Milton Senn, as quoted in "Eleven Years of Love: A Special Tribute to Dr. Arnold S. Anderson," Children's Health Center of Minneapolis, February 1978, 3.
81 Robert Green, *Clini Call*, September, 1967, 3.

Chapter 9

82 Wyman Jacobson, President's Annual Report, St. Louis Park Medical Center, 1969.
83 Glen Nelson, interview with author, August 17, 1994.
84 Arnold Anderson, Minutes of the St. Louis Park Medical Center Board, October 9, 1961.
85 Arnold Anderson, President's Annual Report, St. Louis Park Medical Center, 1963.
86 Glen Nelson, interview with author, August 17, 1994.
87 Loren Vorlicky, Comprehensive Health Care Committee Report, Annual Report of St. Louis Park Medical Center, 1970.
88 Minutes of the St. Louis Park Medical Center Board, September 26, 1972.
89 Minutes of the Medcenter Health Plan, September 5, 1973.
90 Minutes of Medcenter Health Plan Board, July 25, 1980.
91 Minutes of the St. Louis Park Medical Center Board, October 10, 1971.

92 Minutes of the St. Louis Park Medical Center Board, September 26, 1972. Actual date of the opening was September 18, 1972.
93 Glen Nelson, Minutes of the St. Louis Park Medical Center Board, November 12, 1974.
94 Robert Jensen, Annual Report of St. Louis Park Medical Center, 1974.
95 James Stolhanske, Annual Report of St. Louis Park Medical Center, 1979.
96 Norman Sterrie, President's Annual Report, St. Louis Park Medical Center, 1971.
97 Glen Nelson, Annual Reports of St. Louis Park Medical Center, 1972 and 1973.
98 Minutes of the St. Louis Park Medical Center Board, November 3, 1981.
99 Minutes of the St. Louis Park Medical Center Board, October 5, 1982.

Chapter 10
100 St. Louis Park Medical Center Research Foundation Prospectus, 1961, 4.
101 Arnold Anderson et al., eds., *Cerebral Dysfunction: A Community Approach to This School Problem of Children* (Proceedings of conference sponsored by the Richfield Public Schools and St. Louis Park Medical Center Research Foundation, January 16, 1961), 1.
102 Arnold Anderson, Annual Report of St. Louis Park Medical Center, 1964.
103 William Fifer, Annual Report of St. Louis Park Medical Center, 1968.
104 "Professional-courtesy patients" refers to colleagues in the medical profession and their families to whom St. Louis Park Medical Center physicians gave free medical care.
105 Annual Report of Park Nicollet Medical Center, 1984.
106 Arnold Anderson, President's Annual Report, St. Louis Park Medical Center, 1963.
107 Minutes of the St. Louis Park Medical Center Board, May 14, 1974. A review of the report compiled by the "Ten-Clinic Club."
108 Glen Nelson, interview with author, August 17, 1994, and written responses, August 17, 1994.
109 J. Roger Asplin, Administrator's Annual Report, St. Louis Park Medical Center, 1975.
110 Paul Batalden, Annual Report of the St. Louis Park Medical Center Research Foundation, 1982.
111 Annual Report of the St. Louis Park Medical Center Research Foundation, 1979-80.

112 Paul Batalden, President's Report, St. Louis Park Medical Center Research Foundation, 1983.
113 Minutes of Park Nicollet Medical Center, August 23, 1983.
114 "IDC Opening," *What's News?*, October 14, 1983, 1.
115 Minutes of Park Nicollet Medical Center Executive Committee, April 11, 1984.
116 Minutes of Park Nicollet Medical Center, May 27, 1986.
117 Minutes of Medcenter Health Plan Board, January 24, 1975.
118 Annual Report of St. Louis Park Medical Center, 1977.
119 Richard Reeves, "An Interview with Glen Nelson," *Minnesota Medicine* 69(June 1986): 333.
120 A. Stuart Hanson Proposal, Minutes of the St. Louis Park Medical Center Board, December 26, 1978.
121 SHAPE, Annual Report of St. Louis Park Medical Center, 1981.
122 James Reinertsen, Minutes of the St. Louis Park Medical Center Board, April 24, 1979.
123 "Quality Staff Cited as Key to SHAPE Success," *What's News?*, July 13, 1984, 1.
124 Merger Documents of Park Nicollet Medical Center, 1983.

Chapter 11
125 John LaBree, Internal Medicine Annual Report, St. Louis Park Medical Center, 1963.
126 *Clini Call*, August 31, 1964.
127 Minutes of the St. Louis Park Medical Center Board, March 17, 1970.
128 "Residency Program Initiated at Medical Center," *Clini Call*, June 1967, 1.
129 Earl Young, "Objectives and Responsibilities of the Surgical Residency Program," *Clini Call*, June 1967, 1.
130 Cecil Watson, *Outlines of Internal Medicine*, 9th ed. (Dubuque, Iowa: William C. Brown Publishers, 1958).
131 "Answer to MD's Eliminating Long Hard Routine...," *Medical Tribune*, June 19, 1965, 8.
132 William Fifer, Medical Education Report, Minutes of the St. Louis Park Medical Center Research Foundation, June 1969.
133 Francis Foote Manning, ed., *Medical Group Practice Management* (Cambridge, Mass.: Center for Research in Ambulatory Health Care Administration, 1977).
134 Minutes of the St. Louis Park Medical Center Board, February 10, 1958.
135 Arnold Anderson, Minutes of the St. Louis Park Medical Center Board, January 15, 1959.

136 Arnold Anderson, President's Annual Report, St. Louis Park Medical Center,1961.
137 Robert Benjamin, "The Sympathetic Clinic," *Clini Call*, January 15, 1962, 1.
138 J. Roger Asplin, "From the Administrator," *Clini Call*, June 1967, 2.
139 Wyman Jacobson, "The Accreditation of Medical Clinics," (Keynote address presented to the American Association of Medical Clinics, New Orleans, September 26, 1968; published in *Group Practice*, January 1969, 29).
140 Minutes St. Louis Park Medical Center, January 28, 1975, a comment recorded during the discussion of Paul Batalden's proposal to come to work at the clinic.
141 Paul Batalden and J. Paul O'Connor, "Interstudy Fourth Annual Report to the W. K. Kellogg Foundation," Quality Assurance Program, St. Louis Park Medical Center, August 1979, 28.
142 Paul Batalden and J. Paul O'Connor, *Quality Assurance in Ambulatory Care* (Germantown, Md.: Aspen System Corp, 1980): citing work by R. I. Lee and L. W. Jones, *The Fundamentals of Good Medical Care* (Chicago: University of Chicago Press, 1933), 1:3.
143 Batalden and O'Connor, "Interstudy Fourth Annual Report to the W. K. Kellogg Foundation," 9.
144 Linda Zimmey, Paul Batalden et. al, "Patient Telephone Interviews: A Valuable Technique for Finding Problems and Assessing Quality in Ambulatory Medical Care," *The Journal of Community Health* 6(Fall 1980): 36.
145 Ibid.
146 Paul Batalden and J. Paul O'Connor, "Final Report to the Kellogg Foundation," St. Louis Park Medical Center Research Foundation, Health Services Research Center, August 1982.
147 Ibid.
148 Paul Batalden, Annual Report of St. Louis Park Medical Center, 1981.
149 Paul Batalden, Annual Report of St. Louis Park Medical Center, 1982.
150 Odin Anderson et al, *HMO Development: Patterns and Prospects: A Comparative Analysis of HMOs* (Chicago: Pluribus Press, 1985), 283.
151 Robert Green, Minutes of St. Louis Park Medical Center, January 14, 1980.
152 A. Stuart Hanson, Annual Report of St. Louis Park Medical Center, 1980.

Photo History
Part 2

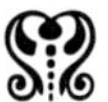

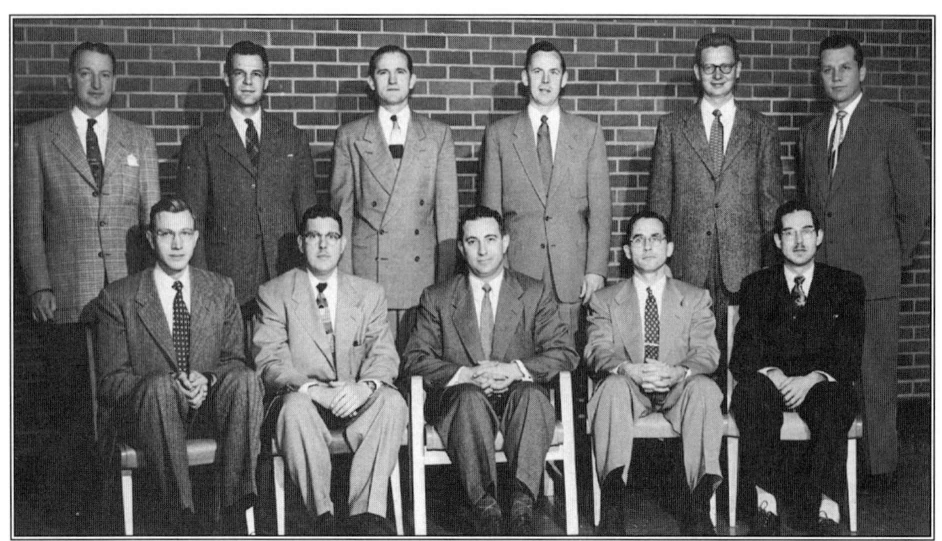

FOUNDERS OF THE ST. LOUIS PARK MEDICAL CENTER, JULY 2, 1951
Front row (l to r): George Lund, Pediatrics; Wyman Jacobson, Internal Medicine; Sewell Gordon, Radiology; Robert "Bud" Green, Internal Medicine; David Anderson, Urology. Back row (l to r): Richard Webber, General Surgery; Robert Giebink, Orthopedics; Alex Barno, Obstetrics/Gynecology; John LaBree, Internal Medicine; Arnold Anderson, Pediatrics; and Donald Freeman, Obstetrics/Gynecology
Photo circa 1951

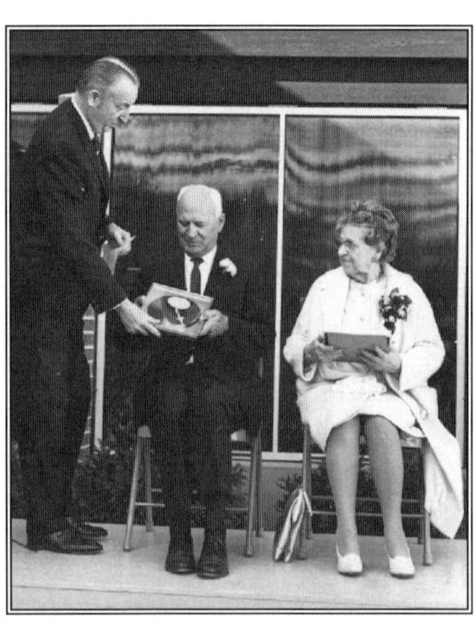

The generosity of Morten and Katheren Arneson changed the futures of the eleven founders. In 1968 the medical center's original building, built on the site of the Arneson's landscape nursery, was dedicated as the "Arneson Building," and the couple was presented gold commemorative keys. "You held the keys to our future, and you hold the keys to our heart," said Dr. Richard Webber.
Photo circa 1968

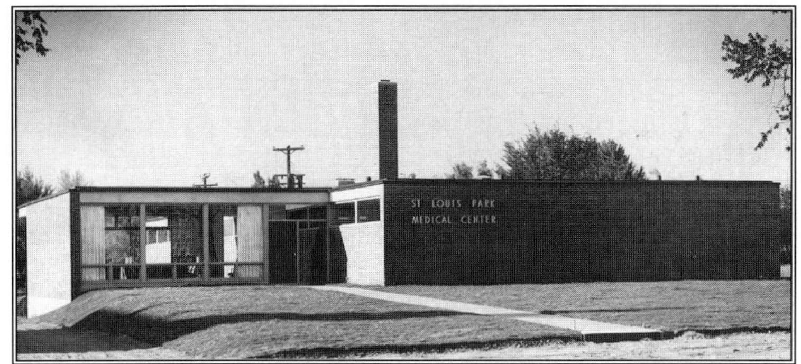

The concept of the St. Louis Park Medical Center was born in 1949 when a young physician named Richard Webber gathered ten other physicians to form a "group practice," a relatively unknown concept at the time.

On July 2, 1951, the St. Louis Park Medical Center opened its doors at 4959 Excelsior Boulevard.

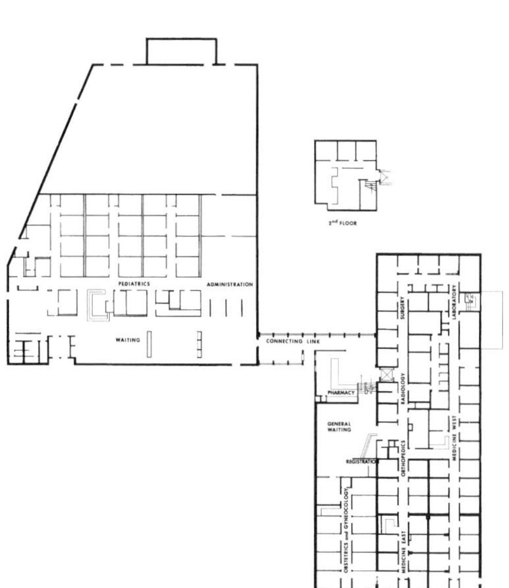

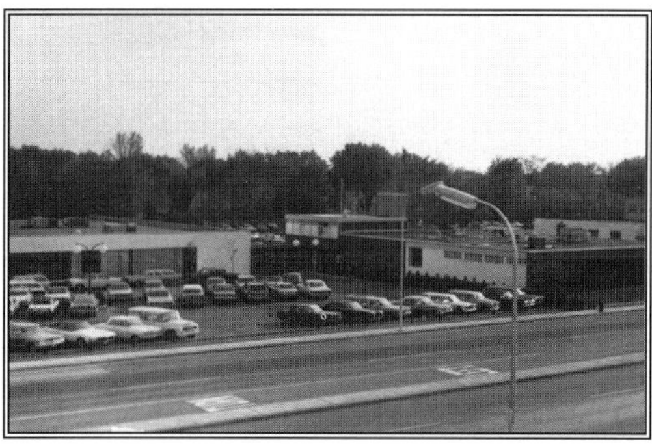

Almost from the beginning, the St. Louis Park Medical Center facility was bursting at the seams. An expansion plan in 1965 involved converting the next-door grocery store into a state-of-the-art pediatrics department, connecting it to the original building by a heated corridor.
Photo circa 1971, facing south across Excelsior Boulevard

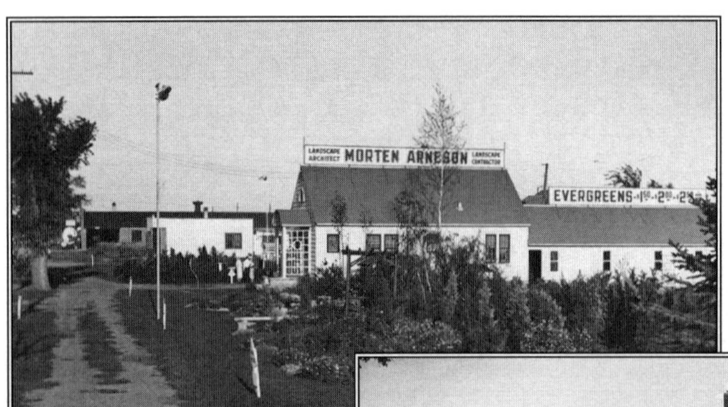

A—*Arneson Nursery, circa 1940s*

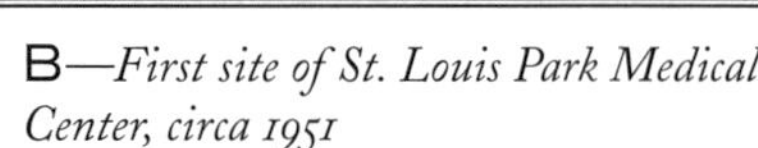

B—*First site of St. Louis Park Medical Center, circa 1951*

C—*Miracle Mile Shopping Center*
Photo circa 1955, Norton & Peel Photography; courtesy of the Minnesota Historical Society

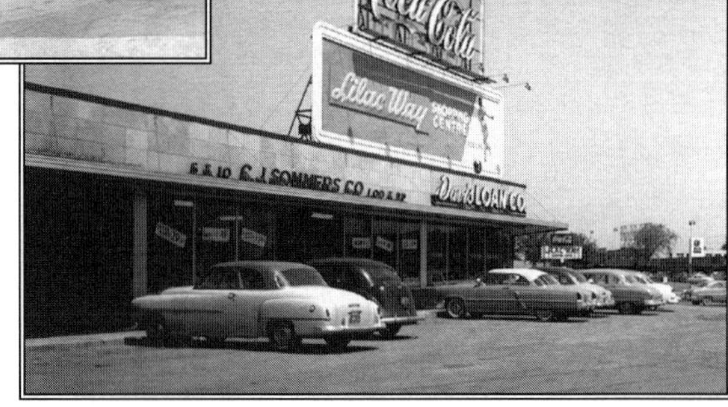

D—*Lilac Way Shopping Center*
Photo circa 1953, Norton & Peel Photography; courtesy of the Minnesota Historical Society

E—*The St. Louis Park Medical Center's "Northland Building" was built at this site in 1969*

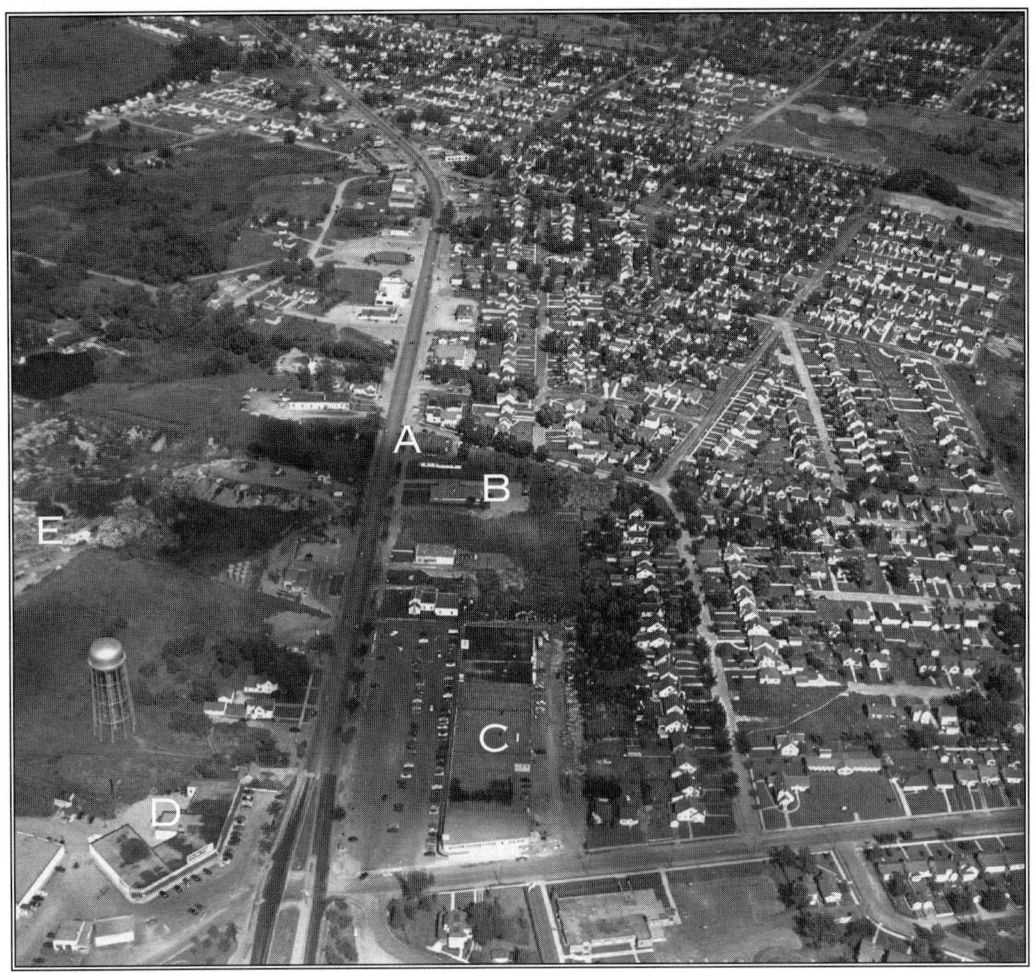

Between 1940 and 1950, St. Louis Park changed dramatically from a rural landscape to a burgeoning suburb. The population had almost tripled in size, from 7,700 in 1940 to 23,000 in 1950. Spurred on by this rapid growth, city planners wanted to develop this stretch of Excelsior Boulevard into a downtown. This aerial view is facing east over Excelsior Boulevard, with Route (Highway) 100 just off the bottom of the photo. Photo circa 1951, Minneapolis StarTribune; courtesy of the Minnesota Historical Society

E
N S
W

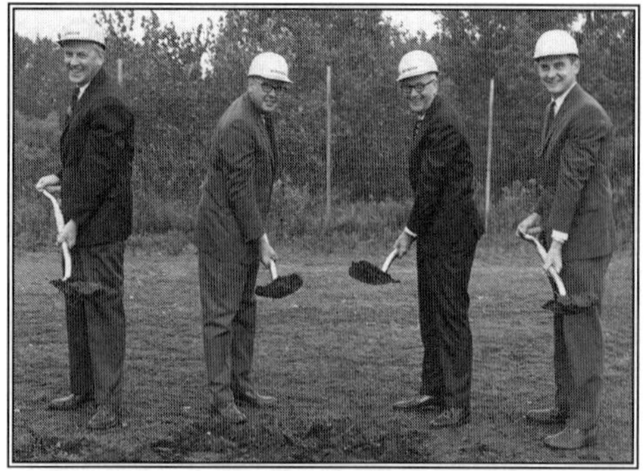

The ground breaking ceremony for the St. Louis Park Medical Center's new six-story building included Dr. Norman A. Sterrie, chairman of the building committee; Dr. Wyman E. Jacobson, president of the St. Louis Park Medical Center Trust; J. Roger Asplin; and Dr. Clyde K. Kitchen, board member of Medcenter, Inc., which owned the physical facilities. Photo circa 1967

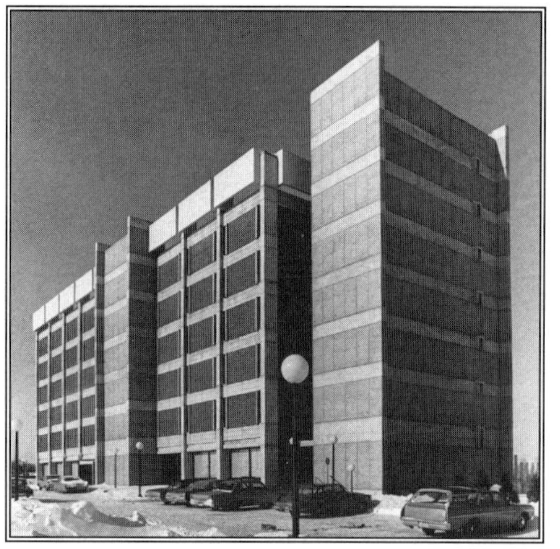

The St. Louis Park Medical Center's new "Northland Building," as it came to be called, was dedicated on January 18, 1969. Located across the street from the original site, the impressive facility had ample room for patient parking and future growth.
Photo circa 1969

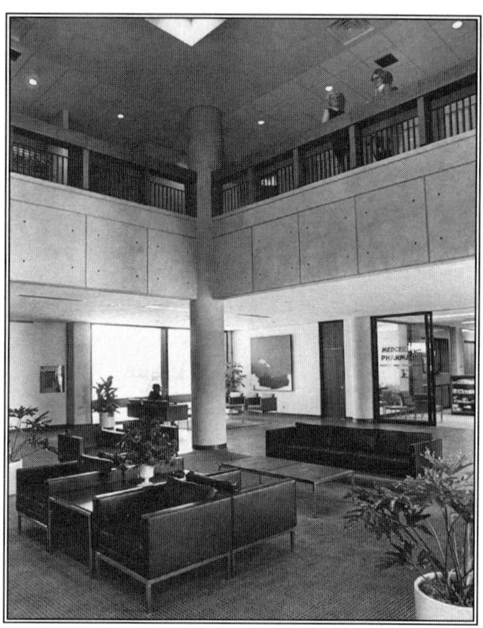

The lobby of the Northland Building, circa 1969

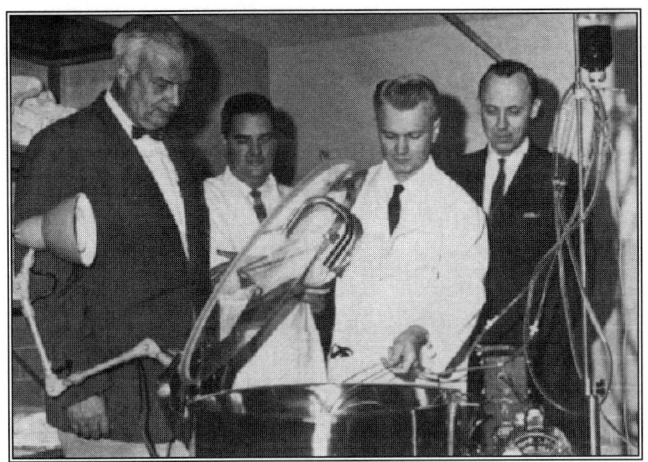

Patients suffering from acute kidney failure got a second chance at life in 1962 when Methodist Hospital purchased an "artificial kidney," one of only two such machines in Minnesota at the time. A young physician, Donald A. Duncan, became the director of the Methodist Hospital program upon joining the St. Louis Park Medical Center in 1962. Pictured inspecting the new machine are (l to r): Vernon T. Spry, Dr. Edward Segal, Dr. Donald Duncan, and Clifford Retherford.
Photo circa 1962; courtesy of Suburban Newspapers

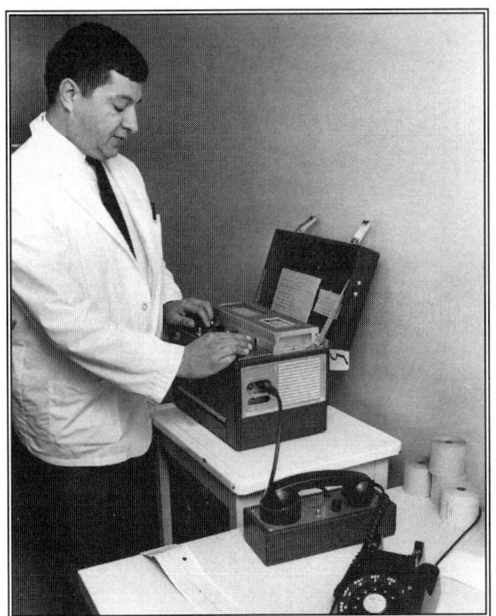

The "heart line" service provided round the clock consulting services, serving hospitals in out-lying areas that did not have cardiologists. The electrocardiogram was transmitted through telephone lines to a team of six medical center physicians who screened for emergency cases. Cardiology technician Nat Flores is seen operating the service.
Photo circa 1969

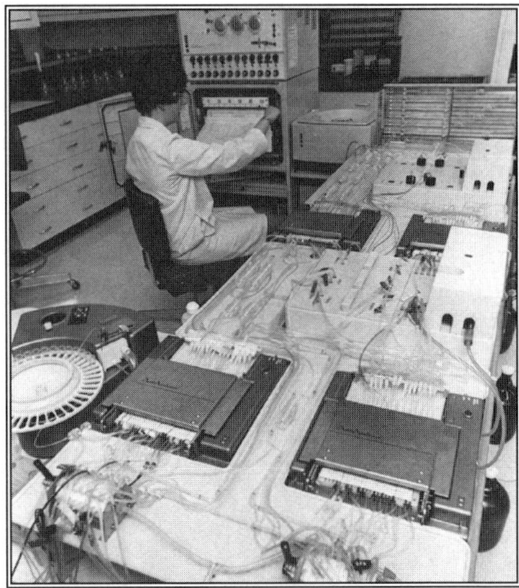

New laboratory equipment at St. Louis Park Medical Center included this $32,000 Sequential Multiple Analyzer which ran twelve chemical blood serum tests in ten minutes. Pictured reading the results is Judyth Larson, medical laboratory assistant.
Photo circa 1969

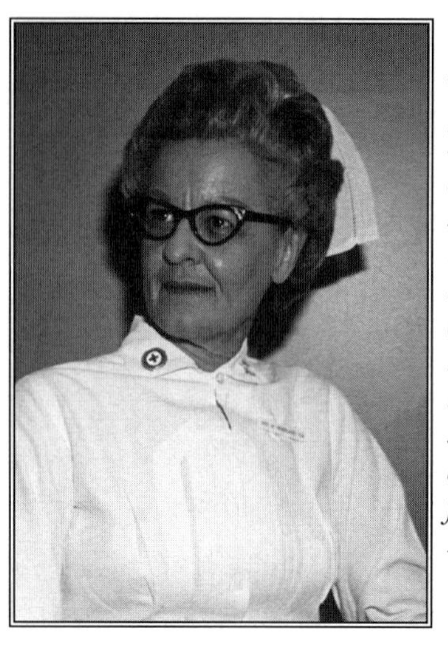

"Help comes with a personal touch for patients at St. Louis Park clinic," the Minneapolis Tribune *headline proclaimed in December, 1971. Registered nurse Cassell Wherland lent a personal touch to callers by patiently hearing their stories and assisting them in choosing a doctor, setting up appointments, and estimating medical fees.*
Photo circa 1971

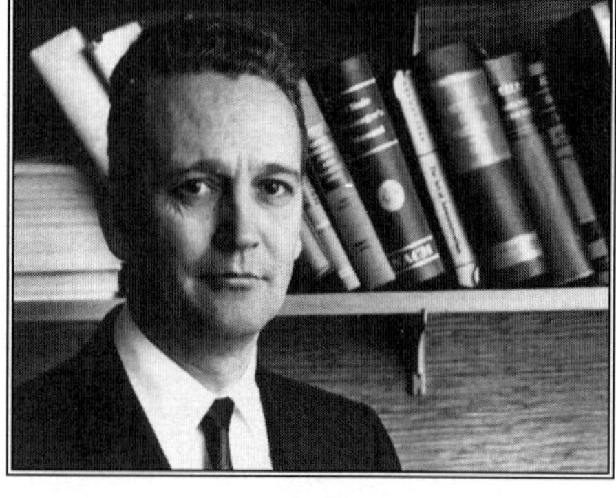

J. Roger Asplin, whose employment at St. Louis Park Medical Center spanned 1958 to 1982, was instrumental in the medical center's growth and in its education and research programs.
Photo circa 1970s

St. Louis Park Medical Center's First Satellite Clinics

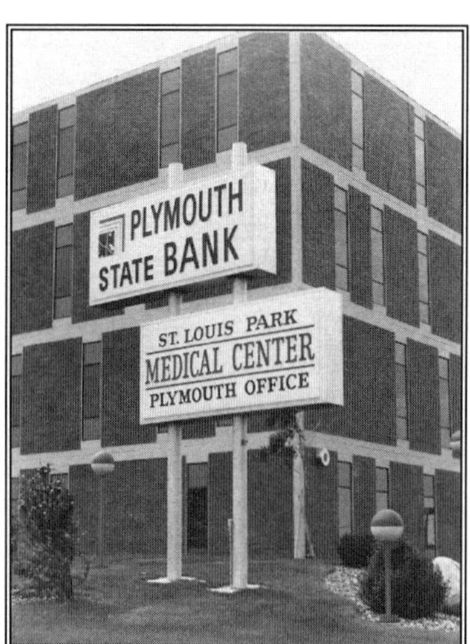

To avoid antagonizing suburban physicians, the St. Louis Park Medical Center studied demographics of surrounding suburbs to find those communities with few or no physicians. One such area was Plymouth, where the first satellite opened in September 1972.

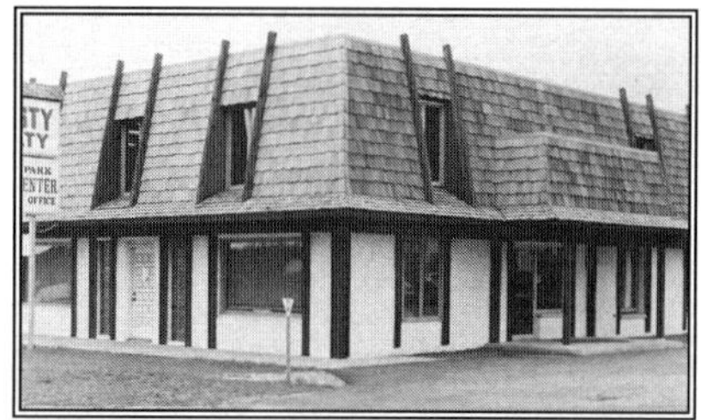

In August 1974, the Minnetonka office opened in the Christy Building at the corner of Highways 101 and 7 under the leadership of Dr. Donald Pine.

In January 1975, the office of Dr. Floyd Swenson, located near the Ridgedale Shopping Center in Minnetonka, joined the medical center's satellite system.

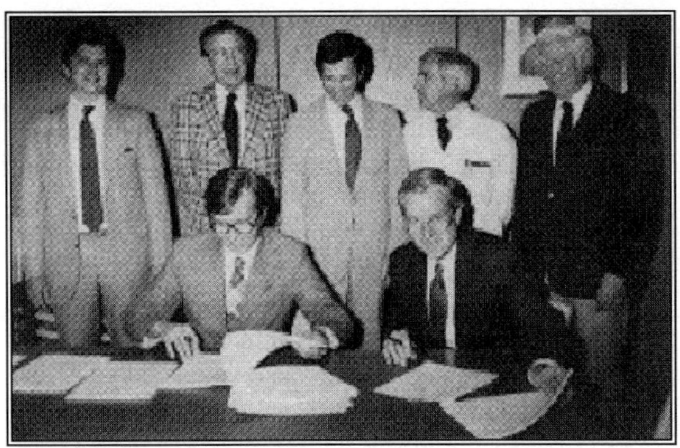

Talk of a merger between St. Louis Park Medical Center and the Nicollet Clinic began in the early 1980s, and on May 25, 1983, a formal agreement was reached. Though the two organizations seemed similar, they had distinct identities and very different traditions. Consequently, the merger was both painful and advantageous for both organizations.

The formal signing of the merger agreement included: (seated) Dr. Paul Batalden, executive vice-president for medical management, and Dr. Glen Nelson, president and chief executive officer; and (l to r) David Lilly, legal counsel; Dr. Thomas M. Recht, associate executive vice-president for professional management; James G. Stolhanske, senior administrator for the St. Louis Park Medical Center; Dr. Loren Vorlicky, chairman and medical director of MedCenters Health Plan; and William Costello, senior administrator for the Nicollet Clinic.

The new organization, named Park Nicollet, offered the services of 210 physicians and more than 1,150 support people in 13 medical offices in Minneapolis. It was now one of the largest group practices in the country.

Park Nicollet Mission

- To promote and maintain the highest standards of compassionate personal care and medical proficiency in the physician-patient relationship;

- To preserve the individual identities of all members of the group and, at the same time, share their resources and experience with the group for mutual benefit and for the benefit of all who come to us for medical care;

- To reflect credit on the communities in which we work and live and, by maintaining the highest standards in our practice of medicine, contribute to the health and enrich the lives of those around us; and

- To contribute individually and together to the advancement of medical science through research and education and to the improvement of systems of health care delivery for the benefit of all.

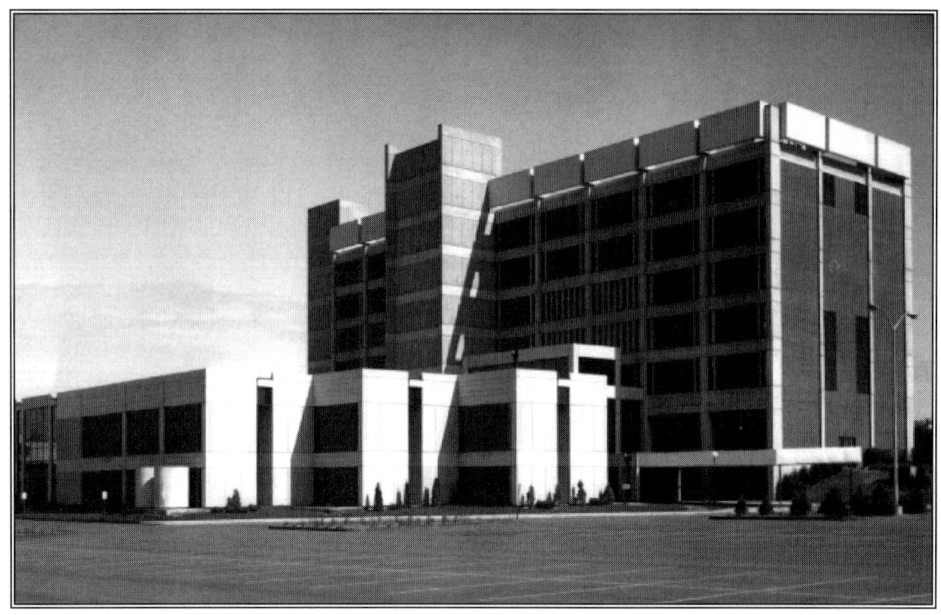

Due to continued dramatic growth, the St. Louis Park Medical Center had built an addition to the north side of the existing building in 1978. The new "Arneson Pavillion," named after Morten and Katheren Arneson, allowed for the geographic consolidation of all clinical departments. The North Tower, designed to house the International Diabetes Center and add badly needed clinical space, was built atop the Arneson Pavillion in 1983 (see photo opposite).
Photo circa 1978; courtesy of Sun Newspapers

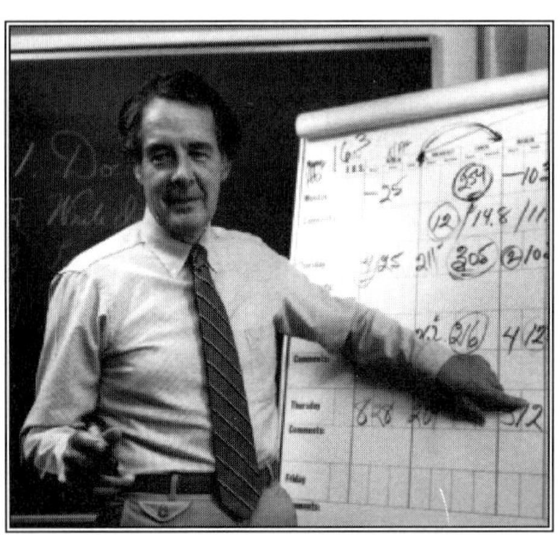

In 1967, pediatrician Donnell D. Etzwiler launched the Diabetes Detection and Education Center with a three-year, $506,000 grant from the Public Health Service. Etzwiler believed that educating patients to participate in their care was key to successful diabetes control.

The center eventually became part of the St. Louis Park Medical Research Foundation and had, by the early 1980s, outgrown its cramped quarters. To fund the North Tower construction, the foundation began the medical center's most impressive capital campaign yet. The diabetes center was renamed International Diabetes Center in 1983.

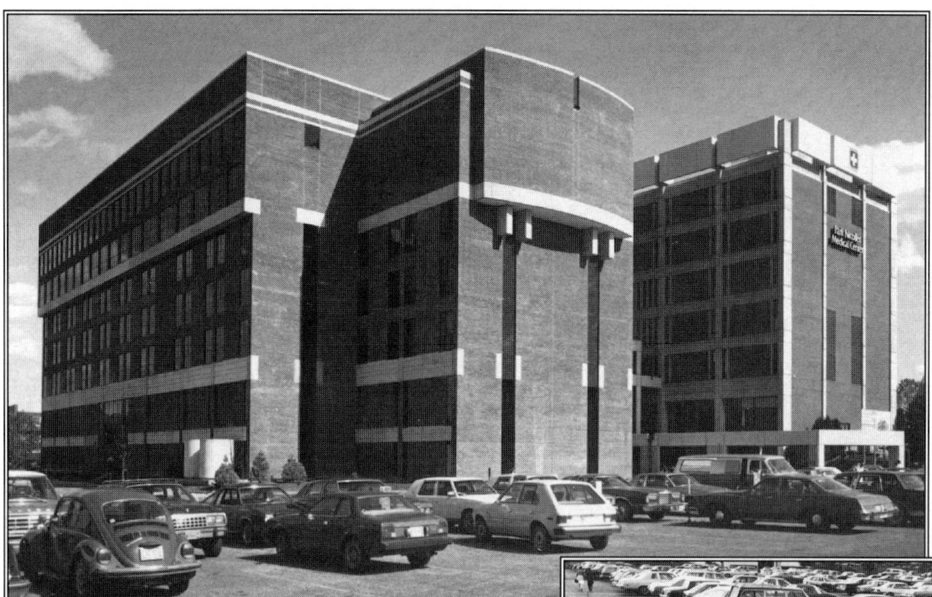

Under the leadership of James V. Toscano, vice president of the St. Louis Park Medical Research Foundation, the capital campaign to build a suitable location for the International Diabetes Center was an exciting but challenging endeavor.

In the same year that St. Louis Park Medical Center and the Nicollet Clinic merged, the groundbreaking for the North Tower took place. Minnesota's Governor Rudy Perpich was in attendance on October 12, 1983, and he declared the day "International Diabetes Center Day in Minnesota."

By the time the tower was dedicated on September 7, 1985, the total project cost had topped $15.5 million, about $10 million of which had been raised from the community.

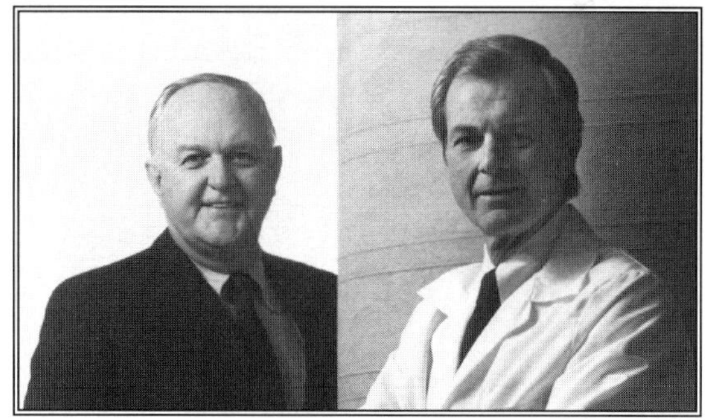

Dale Olseth, president of Medtronic, Inc., and Dr. Glen D. Nelson, president of St. Louis Park Medical Center, co-chaired the fund-raising committee for the North Tower construction.
Photo circa 1983

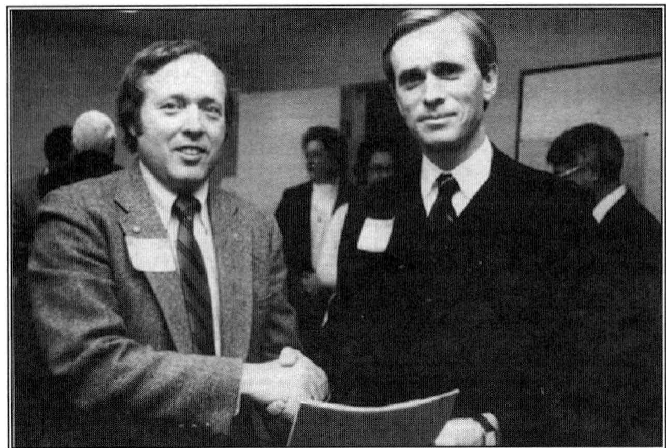

On January 15, 1985, a final merger agreement was reached between Skakopee Medical Center and Park Nicollet. The Skakopee Medical Center's affiliate clinic, the Prior Lake Health Center, was also part of the merger. Pictured here are Dr. Donald Abrams, (left), president of Shakopee Medical Center, and Dr. James Reinertsen, trustee of Park Nicollet.
Photo circa 1985

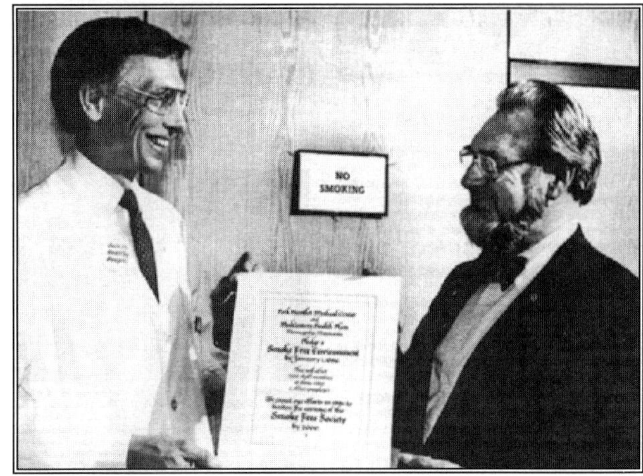

Dr. A. Stuart Hanson presented a declaration to Dr. C. Everett Koop, United States Surgeon General, during a ceremony at Park Nicollet on March 13, 1985. The declaration pledged that the medical center would become smoke-free by January 1, 1986.
Photo circa 1985

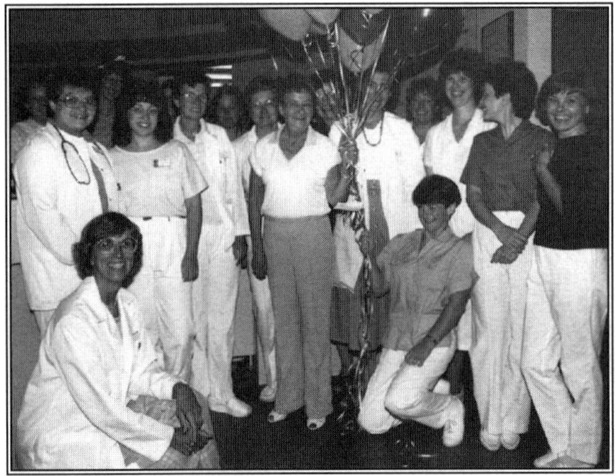

Jean Tollefson (Beardsley), the first secretary at the St. Louis Park Medical Center in 1952, is pictured here (holding balloons) celebrating her retirement with her Plymouth Clinic colleagues in 1987. She left the medical center in 1956 to raise her children, but returned to the organization in 1973.
Photo circa 1987

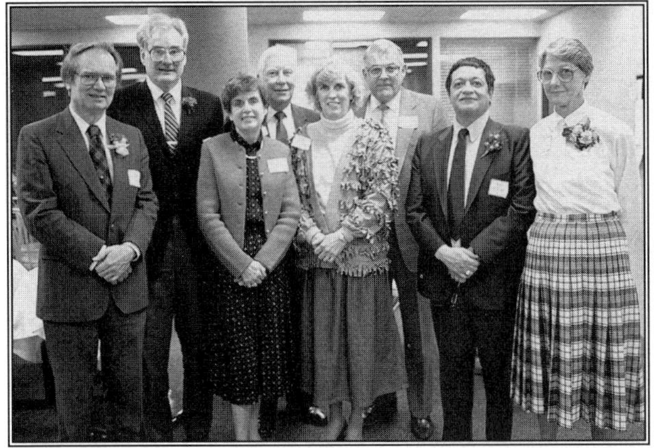

Some of the employees honored for twenty five and thirty years of service include (l to r): Drs. Donald Duncan, Richard Woellner, and Jeanne Bradley; William Costello; Ruth Lee; Dr. John Powers; Nat Flores; and Margaret Clemmings.
Photo circa 1988

The Park Nicollet Corporate Volunteer Council organized employee involvement in the annual Paint-a-Thon, a program sponsored by the Greater Minneapolis Council of Churches.
Photo circa 1988

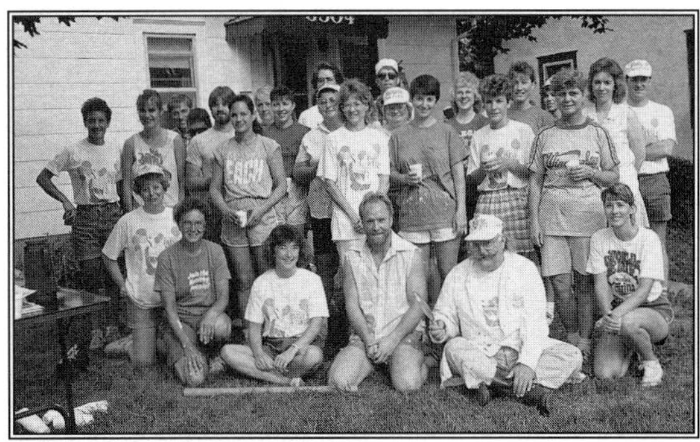

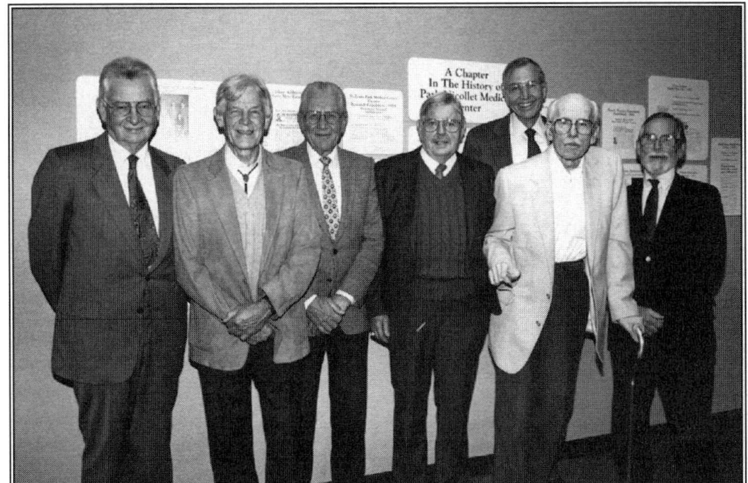

Seven of the eleven founding physicians of St. Louis Park Medical Center stood in front of the exhibit that documents the medical center's beginning. (l to r): Arnold Anderson; Robert Giebink; Donald Freeman; Wyman Jacobson; George Lund; Alex Barno; and Robert (Bud) Green.
Photo circa 1988

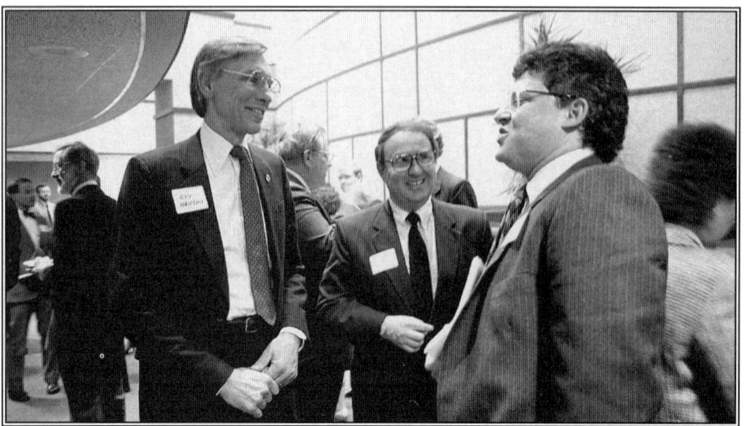

Dr. A. Stuart Hanson, (left) chairman of Park Nicollet Medical Foundation, and James V. Toscano, (center) executive vice president, visited with Arthur Caplan, Ph.D., director of the Biomedical Ethics Center at the University of Minnesota. Caplan was the featured speaker at the foundation's 1988 annual meeting. His presentation was on the rationing of health care, government policy, and desired responses in the medical community.
Photo circa 1988

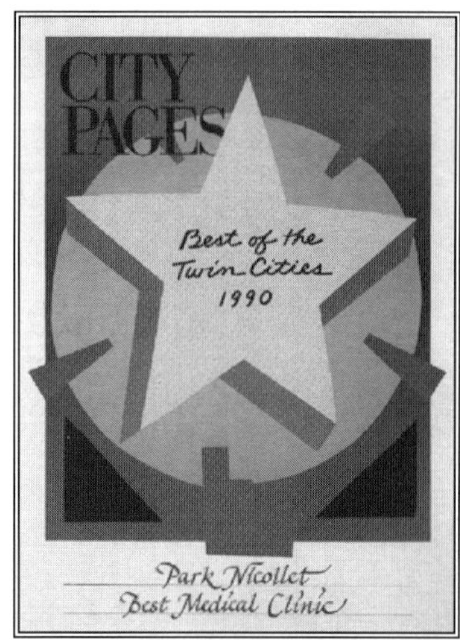

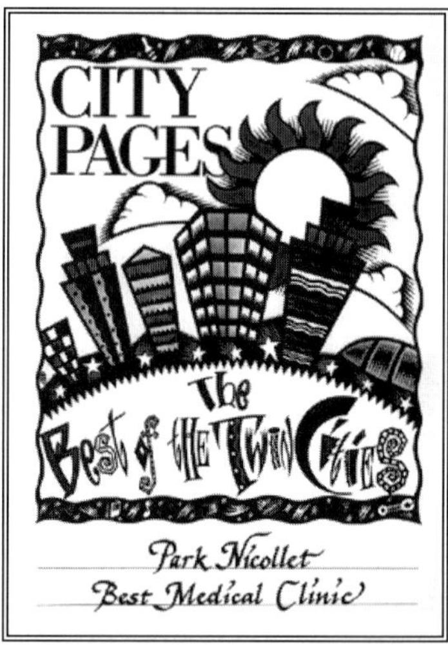

Park Nicollet was voted "Best Medical Clinic in the Twin Cities" by City Pages *readers in 1990 and 1991, and it was voted into the newspaper's "Hall of Fame" in 1994.*

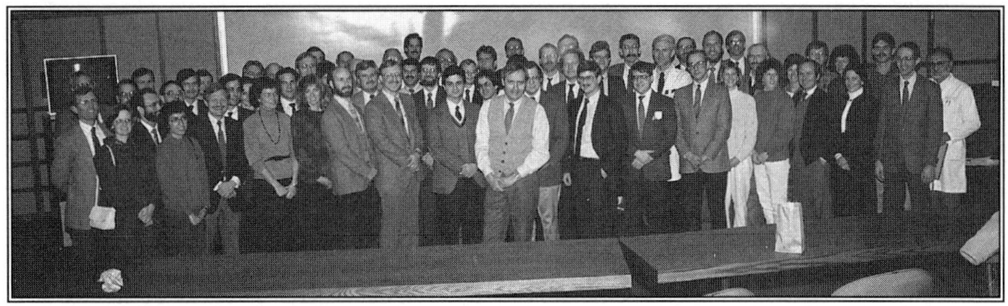

Park Nicollet staff gathered to honor Dr. Allan Kind (in center) for his work as medical director. He is surrounded by the many physicians who were hired during his tenure.
Photo circa 1988

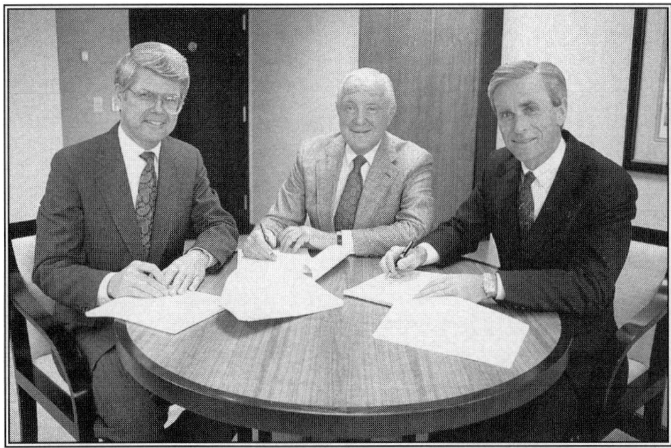

The establishment of the first major physician-hospital affiliation in the Twin Cities was the first step toward integrating inpatient and outpatient services into a true system of care.

On December 11, 1991, Joseph W. Mitlyng, Park Nicollet senior vice president and chief operating officer, Robert Galloway, Methodist president and chief executive officer, and Dr. James L. Reinertsen, Park Nicollet president and chief executive officer, put an agreement on paper that led to the formation of HealthSystem Minnesota in 1993.
Photo circa 1992

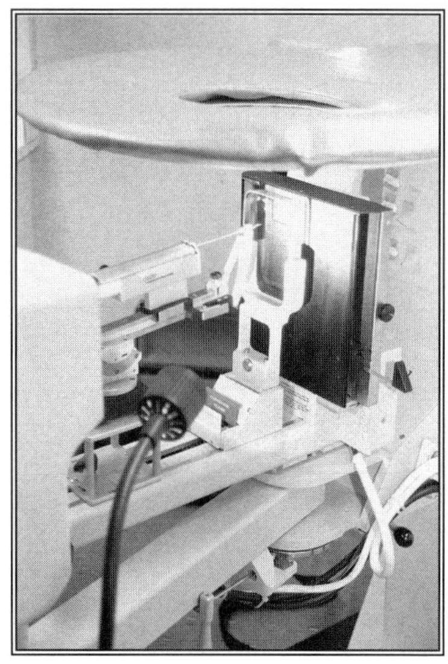

Maintaining its tradition of state-of-the-art medical technology, Park Nicollet installed this breast biopsy equipment—the first of its kind in the Twin Cities metropolitan area—in 1992. The technology, known as Mammotest, is designed to locate small breast lesions and collect tissue samples for analysis.
Photo circa 1992

HealthSystem Minnesota

In 1993 Methodist Hospital, Methodist Hospital Foundation (now The Foundation), Park Nicollet (18 clinic locations), and Primary Physician Network (9 clinic locations), formally merged and a parent company, HealthSystem Minnesota, was established. In 1995 the Family Physicians of Northfield joined HealthSystem Minnesota, as did Park Nicollet Medical Foundation (now the Institute for Research and Education) in 1996.

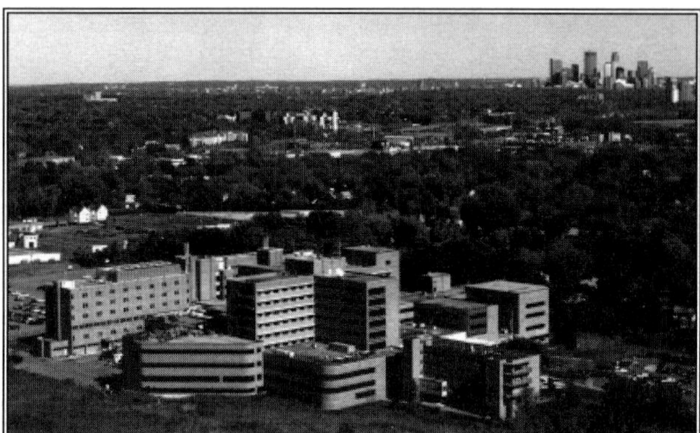

Since 1959, when Asbury Methodist Hospital moved from Minneapolis to St. Louis Park, Methodist Hospital has maintained a vital association with Park Nicollet. This photo, facing east towards downtown Minneapolis, shows the hospital's campus in 1994.

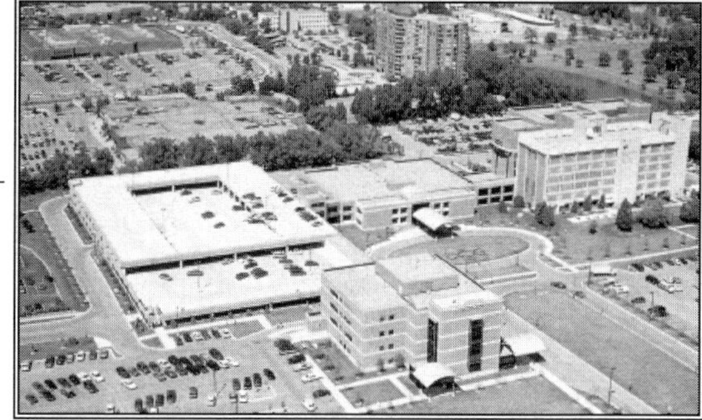

This photo, facing north, shows the expanded campus of the Northland Building as of 1995.

This diamond is a picture of the core values that exemplify HealthSystem Minnesota's vision and strategic intent, "HealthSystem Minnesota will become the care system in which care and service are so good, and costs so low, that our patients and staff will refuse to go elsewhere."

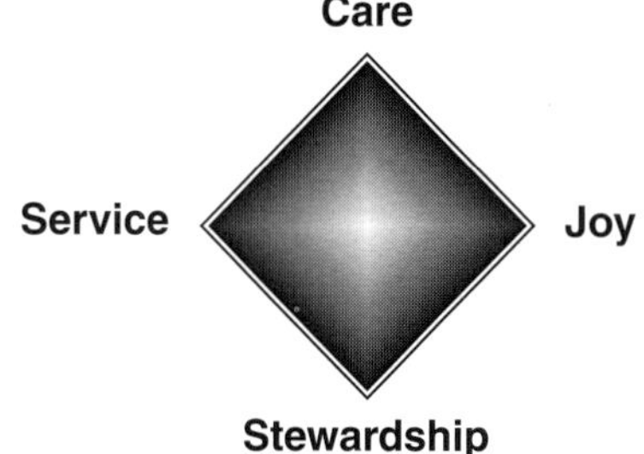

Part Three

Park Nicollet

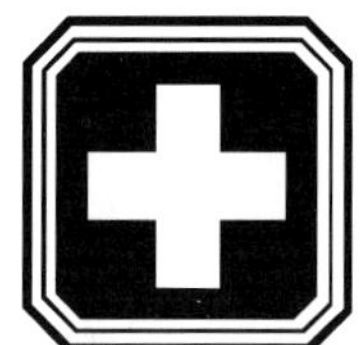

12

JOINING FORCES
THE FOUNDING OF PARK NICOLLET

THE ADVENT OF THE HMO MOVEMENT IN THE EARLY 1970S meant major changes for St. Louis Park Medical Center and the Nicollet Clinic. Both considered themselves, first and foremost, multispecialty, referral clinics. But the economic and market dynamics of the time spurred them to create their own HMOs. This made each group responsible to a set of patients for their primary, secondary, and tertiary care.

The St. Louis Park group, making the most of their larger size, chose to bring a network of primary care providers into their Medcenter Health Plan, sacrificing some control over the health plan for a much-more-rapid growth curve. The Nicollet Clinic and its partner, Eitel Hospital, chose to keep all primary care within the group to maximize their control over the services provided, but they actively sought all the growth that could be generated internally.

Both the Medcenter Health Plan, founded in 1972, and the Nicollet-Eitel Family Health Plan, started in 1973, quickly found ready markets. What both physician groups had envisioned as a tentative experiment—a test of the ability of the HMO to support the development of the group practice—exploded into the market and took on a life of its own. Patient demand for lower-cost medical insurance, which included preventive care and little paper-

"The group's efficient use of the total health care dollar was unmasked by the prepayment mechanism."[2]

Glen Nelson, M.D., 1982
Competition in the Marketplace

work, made any retreat from the new HMOs inconceivable after only a few months of operation.

In the new market, with health plans competing for the same large employee groups, the ability to offer convenient access to clinical services across a broad geographic region became a major marketing advantage. A patient referred by his or her local private practice physician might be happy to go to a central office for specialty care, but the healthy people who signed up for health plans wanted to go to a neighborhood clinic for routine care. Employers screening health care plans were looking closely at geographic accessibility. It was a market signal impossible to ignore, and both groups responded by opening suburban satellite clinics. "People aren't sick when they sign up," Glen Nelson explained, "so they ask: 'Is the office convenient, and is the price right?' They don't say: 'If I were really sick, I wouldn't mind driving across town to get to the best doctors.'"

COMPETITION

For the first few years the Medcenter and Nicollet-Eitel health plans had little outside competition. Both were attracting subscribers from specific geographic areas. Both were attractively priced, compared with the indemnity plans. Both tended to attract young, healthy people who had not already established important relationships with individual physicians, and people who were already patients of the clinics.[1] More importantly, both clinics ordered fewer hospital-bed days per patient than the community average, virtually assuring their financial viability. St. Louis Park Medical Center, for instance, was using 400 bed days per 1,000 patients in 1972, compared with the community average of between 800 and 900.

Although, technically, the two health plans were competing with each other for members, there was little sense of this during the first years of operation. Northwestern National Life, the marketing agent for the Medcenter Health Plan, also offered the Nicollet-Eitel Family Health Plan to its employer groups, a fact that seemed to concern no one at the time. The executive directors of the two HMOs, Nick Spring of Nicollet-Eitel and Steve Goldstone of Medcenter, had been classmates at the University of Minnesota.[3] In 1973, they discussed possible joint marketing efforts, but there had been little interest at either clinic for these business office ideas as market conditions were highly favorable to the two group-practice HMOs at the time.

By the mid-1970s, competition for health plan subscribers in the Twin Cities metropolitan area had heated up. In addition to Group Health, the largest of the existing plans, Blue Cross Blue Shield of Minnesota and the Hennepin County Medical Society unveiled their own HMO products, HMO Minnesota and Physicians Health Plan respectively. Tom Hobban, the director of the Hennepin County Medical Society, remembered this was at least in part a defensive move "to combat the Nicollet Clinic and St. Louis Park Medical Center who were moving into prepaid care."[4] The new HMOs offered many of the same benefits as the clinic plans with fewer restrictions on the patient's choice of physician. Growth was rapid.

However, by 1976 the Nicollet-Eitel Family Health Plan found itself facing slower growth and rising costs. The decision to control primary care services, combined with the location of the Nicollet Clinic and Eitel Hospital, generated a membership in the Nicollet-Eitel plan that was largely urban, older, and single—all characteristics pointing to higher costs, "adverse selection" in the jargon of health insurance. As evidence of this adverse selection became more obvious, the Nicollet-Eitel plan and the Nicollet Clinic began to look seriously at available options for strategic alliances that could broaden the plan's appeal and improve its finances.

Charles Bredesen, who formerly had been in charge of

marketing the Medcenter Health Plan for Northwestern National Life, was brought in as a consultant to help revitalize the Nicollet-Eitel Family Health Plan. Among his many suggestions was the exploration of a merger of the two health plans. With the Nicollet Clinic's blessing, Bredesen presented the idea to Glen Nelson, president of St. Louis Park Medical Center, and Loren Vorlicky, medical director of Medcenter Health Plan. Interested, St. Louis Park Medical Center studied the proposal and decided that the primary market advantage of such a merger could be generated only if the two clinic groups were merged as well. But again, the market advantage to be gained was insufficient to convince a majority of physicians at either clinic to make the changes a merger would require, and the discussions ended.

LOOKING FOR A STRATEGIC PARTNER

If the medical marketplace had suggested a merger in 1976, this same "invisible hand" was demanding it by 1980. Competition for the health care dollar had increased dramatically. New, low-cost, preferred provider organizations were being organized to compete for the healthy young. Unionization of traditionally low-wage nursing and medical support workers was putting pressure on hospitals and clinics alike. The hospitals were under additional pressure to cut the number of excess beds in the Twin Cities area, which according to a Citizens League analysis numbered over four thousand.[5] The vacant beds were perversely creating bed shortages in more popular hospitals, which were prevented by cost-control legislation from building additional space while excess beds existed in the community. These popular hospitals were, in response, refusing entry to new physicians.

It was under these conditions that St. Louis Park Medical Center assented to a proposal from the SHARE organization in St. Paul to consider a merger of the two clinics and associated health plans in April 1980. With 38,000 members, the SHARE Health Plan was roughly half the size of the Medcenter Health Plan. A staff model HMO, SHARE had grown rapidly from only 300 members in 1974.[6] An alliance between SHARE and St. Louis Park Medical Center was appealing, Glen Nelson pointed out, as a way to "gain sufficient critical mass and scale to compete more effectively in the Twin Cities community."[7] A combined organization would have a geographic reach unmatched by any other group practice plan.

As the discovery process was coming to closure in the spring of 1981, the medical center began to have second thoughts. Reports that SHARE had recorded an unanticipated loss of $600,000 in 1980 made the prospective merger financially more difficult. St. Louis Park Medical Center management, facing a union organizing effort in 1980, was uncomfortable with SHARE physicians' outspoken sympathy for health care unions.[8] In the end, the two physician groups just didn't have the right chemistry, and the talks were suspended in April 1981. St. Louis Park Medical Center continued to search for suitable strategic partners.[9]

MERGER DISCUSSIONS

A little more than a year after the collapse of the SHARE negotiations, Thomas Recht, then the medical director of the Nicollet Clinic, suggested to Glen Nelson that it might be time to "seriously think about a merger" of their organizations. Recht had come to "the altruistic point of view that we had two organizations that were competing for the same turf, the same patient base, both with HMOs—it was just redundant as hell." Donald Velleck, president of the Nicollet Clinic, also saw the need for growth. The clinic, he said, "needed to be larger in the future . . . and we had the choice . . . do it ourselves or merge with others who were similar." The reenergized Nicollet-Eitel Health Plan had, since 1977, been increasingly competitive in the southern suburbs, which was driving a rapid expansion of the Nicollet Clinic's suburban offices in Burnsville, Bloomington, and Eagan. In contrast to the merger discussions in 1976, the new energy had substantially improved the Nicollet Clinic's negotiating position and made the prospect of a merger much more interesting to the leadership at St. Louis Park.

Nelson reported his conversation with Recht to the board in July 1982, and the board quietly authorized administrator James Stolhanske to begin a business analysis of the idea. By December, Stolhanske and William Costello, administrator at the Nicollet Clinic, had concluded that the groups were "highly compatible for merger."[10] "Both systems were beginning to expend a lot of capital to differentiate and develop their health plans," Stolhanske recounted. "You had two well-respected groups who had developed group practice HMOs, and the merger was an opportunity to pool our resources to compete with our natural competitors—Group Health, SHARE, and Physicians Health Plan."

David Jensen, hired to replace Steve Goldstone in 1981 as executive director of Medcenter Health Plan, pointed out that the two clinics' health plans were similar in management style and orientation and that the "Nicollet-Eitel Health Plan is really the only option if merger is a desirable way to achieve short-term growth."[11] Merging the health plans "was the right business thing to do," according to Loren Vorlicky, medical director of Medcenter Health Plan at the time. "We found ourselves increasingly competing with Nicollet-Eitel, and not being able to differentiate ourselves in the marketplace. Both were group-practice based, they offered similar benefits, the price was about the same, and we found ourselves needing to build competitive service areas where they already existed and vice versa." Likewise, Charles Bredesen, executive director of the Nicollet-Eitel Health Plan, saw the advantages of a merger: "As the marketplace was getting more competitive and the clutter of advertising and so forth was increasing, [a merger] seemed to me to be a way to reduce marketing expenditures, clarify your market position, and create some competitive advantage vis-à-vis the other models."

While merger discussions in 1973 and 1976 had begun with the idea of combining only the health plans, discussions in 1982 proceeded differently. "We felt a lot of pressure to move quickly in order to make the transition and get back into the marketplace," James Stolhanske explained. "But if you didn't have the delivery system—the clinics—merged, then what did you have to sell? We never considered merging just the health plans even for one day."

Like the Nicollet Clinic, St. Louis Park Medical Center also saw plenty of reasons to seek a merger in self-defense against an uncertain future. In February 1983, Glen Nelson reported to the board that while the final outcome of the negotiations might be uncertain, the process would, in any case, "certainly help us to understand our own operation better and provide further insights into the external environment." The near future, Nelson predicted, was likely to include many new competitors, including a "realignment of physicians and hospitals to form competitive health care organizations . . . large corporations may internalize much of their health care for their employees and buy additional services 'on bid' . . . [and] national firms could enter our market by buying an existing system. The combination of surplus physicians, new laws, corporate economics, and consumer sociology," he continued, "will combine to promote a physician scramble into organizations which can provide the physician some guarantee of security."[12]

Paul Batalden, then president of the rapidly growing St. Louis Park Medical Center Research Foundation, was asked to head a joint task force in January 1983 to explore the professional issues involved in a merger. He immediately set up a schedule for each of the major decision points and legal issues to be negotiated. "I'm pretty sure that if Batalden hadn't been there managing the thing the merger would never have happened," Loren Vorlicky noted in 1994. Nicollet Clinic Board Member Max Boller agreed. "[Batalden] was a tremendous organizer, and he was right on top of everything. He wanted progress reports. He wanted things to move along, and he was a very good administrator."

Numerous issues, however, might have, and almost did, block the deal. Earl Young wrote Nelson in early 1983 of his "strong ambivalence about the proposed merger." Young, who had for years acted as the respected referee of St. Louis Park Medical Center's Professional Compensation Committee, warned that the "weeding out" that might take place "is always a very difficult thing to do. . . . Professionally," he continued, "it may present . . . extraordinarily difficult problems in some departments."[13]

Nor was the decision to merge an easy one at the Nicollet Clinic. A significant and vocal group of physicians within the clinic were not ready to trade the freedom and control they enjoyed as owners of a smaller group. Although organized as a professional corporation years before, the clinic had retained the flavor of a partnership, operating "more like a benevolent association." These reservations, however, didn't sway the younger physicians who were now in the majority at the clinic and who didn't know yet what they would be missing. But even as the date of the merger vote approached, Max Boller remembered, "We all had the impression that the wheels were coming off." To get the merger back on track, Boller canceled his vacation and "spent the whole week taking Nicollet Clinic physicians to meet one-on-one and two-on-two with St. Louis Park people who were in the merger mode. The big question was always control."

THE TWO CLINICS MERGE

One by one the reservations expressed by various individuals in both groups were dealt with or set aside. The wheels went on turning. With the strong support of Nelson, Batalden, Recht, Boller, and others, the merger soon developed its own momentum. A strong business rationale had been established and, as William Costello put it in 1993, "[Once] you have a solid consensus on a valid and valuable purpose for the merger, you persevere and drive the project along dealing fairly and openly with all the many obstacles."

Following Batalden's plan, four separate votes had to occur before the merger of the clinics and their HMOs was complete. The Nicollet-Eitel Health Plan moved first, voting to merge with Medcenter Health Plan in March 1983. The Medcenter Health Plan Board approved the merger two weeks later. A founding board of the new organization, MedCenters Health Plan, was appointed on March 18, 1983, and the merger of the health plans was legally completed and accepted by the state on May 3, 1983. Eitel Hospital, now a member of the Lifespan organization,[14] chose this time to end its co-sponsorship of the plan, but continued as a provider of hospital services. Loren Vorlicky accepted the position of chair of the board, and David Jensen was appointed chief executive officer of the new organization.

With the merger of the health plans accomplished and last-minute objections addressed, both clinics voted to accept the merger agreement and plan in late May. At a public ceremony on May 25, 1983, Donald Velleck, president of the Nicollet Clinic, and Glen Nelson, president of St. Louis Park Medical Center, signed the preliminary papers merging the two groups. Glen Nelson accepted the position as president of the first combined board.

The merger agreement established committees to sort out the salary and pension differences and to integrate the records and information systems and directed the depart-

When consulted about the upcoming talks, Max Boller thought that a merger would be a "great idea." But he remembers telling Tom Recht that although the merger would be very good for the organization, "'It will never happen . . . because our pension plan is significantly different from theirs, and theirs is a disadvantage to physicians, and the people of this organization will never give up their pension plan.' Well, I was wrong and I was right. We didn't give up our pension plan, but that was the linchpin."

MEDCENTERS HEALTH PLAN FOUNDING BOARD, 1983

Loren N. Vorlicky, M.D., Chair
David A. Jensen, CEO
A. Charles Bredesen III, COO
Max Boller, M.D., Director of Medical Affairs
Glen D. Nelson, M.D., Treasurer
Sharon Collins, Secretary, Control Data Corporation
Warren Becker, Sperry Univac
David Buran, M.D.
John Haugen, M.D.
David Knutzen, General Mills
JoAnne Neher, Consumer Representative
John Raplinger, County Seat Stores
James Sipe, M.D., Coon Rapids Medical Center
Nancy Spannus, Minnetonka Public Schools
Gilbert Westreich, M.D.

ments of each clinic to begin professional integration. This latter directive was implemented in each department with varying degrees of enthusiasm. Several departments, pediatrics and the laboratories, for instance, began working together immediately. The pediatrics departments, led by Theresa Ryan at St. Louis Park Medical Center and Richard Allen at the Nicollet Clinic, scheduled a joint retreat so that their departments could get to know one another and discuss the likely problems involved in combining the two groups. Nicollet Clinic pediatricians joined weekly educational meetings at Methodist Hospital and, after the merger was finalized in August 1983, joined regular departmental meetings. By May 1984, the two groups were sharing a single call schedule.[15] Northrop Beach, long-time head of pediatrics at the Nicollet Clinic who retired in 1983, believed that his department had much to gain from the merger with St. Louis Park Medical Center. "Our pediatricians," he said, "received what I would consider an adequate salary only after the merger."

Other departments, such as obstetrics and gynecology, found the process much more difficult. "Combining the two organizations was a slow and agonizing process," obstetrician Mario Petrini remembered. "Each group tended to guard their prior identity." "Cultural differences" became the most common euphemism for the differences in style, unfulfilled ambitions, and the relative acceptance or nonacceptance of the corporate management style of the new organization.[16] "The hardest job we had administratively," Stolhanske recalled, "was to figure out how to bring the organizations together to be efficient and still recognize a certain amount of autonomy for the two groups. I don't think these were very compatible goals."

There were many opportunities later for second thoughts. Looking back on this period, Paul Batalden noted, "I really underestimated the work that the merger would involve. . . . What looks the same isn't necessarily the same, and even though the organizations looked alike, there were different traditions. What was interesting to me was that there was enough difference in the two organizations so that each of them felt very keenly about their identity and the differences that existed. . . . People were proud of their organizations and they didn't want them to die."

One way the new organization fostered the feeling of relative autonomy was to delay any strict assignment of practice location or styles. Nicollet Clinic physicians, for the most part, continued to use the hospitals they had used before the merger, as did St. Louis Park Medical Center physicians. The two Ridgedale clinics were merged into one location within a year, as were the two Eagan clinics. Otherwise, the satellite clinics retained their original staffs and locations for several years. The business offices were combined under the leadership of James Stolhanske and headquartered in the Northland Building, although it took the next five years to accomplish the integration of the scheduling and billing.

On August 2, 1983, the final merger documents were signed. The new organization—encompassing 210 physicians, more than 1,150 support staff, and 13 medical offices, "one of the largest group practices in the country"—had been created.[17] On August 23 the new board met to adopt a new name and a new mission. Park Nicollet was officially born, and its new mission was:

- To promote and maintain the highest standards of compassionate personal care and medical proficiency in the physician-patient relationship;
- To preserve the individual identities of all members of the group and, at the same time, share their resources and experience with the group for mutual benefit and for the benefit of all who come to us for medical care;
- To reflect credit on the communities in which we work and live and, by maintaining the highest standards in our practice of medicine, contribute to the health and enrich the lives of those around us; and

- To contribute individually and together to the advancement of medical science through research and education and to the improvement of systems of health care delivery for the benefit of all.

"The Nicollet Clinic is beginning a new era," Thomas Recht said in his last annual report as medical director. "Some of our traditions will change, some will continue. Regardless, we as an organization have recognized that change is occurring at an accelerated rate and we have had the foresight and courage to meet that challenge. . . . The formation of the new Park Nicollet Medical Center is our response to the future."[18]

Reviewing the status of the combined organization in early 1984, President Glen Nelson reiterated his belief that "larger, vertically integrated organizations will dominate the health care delivery field" and noted that Park Nicollet had managed to "add exceptional human resources and develop new programs," even as "much of our organizational energy was consumed by the merger." Indeed, during 1983 two new satellite clinics were opened, the home care department started operations, the on-site Senior Care Program at Walker Methodist Health Center was opened, and a rehabilitative medicine initiative got underway. This "remarkable strength" was just one indicator of "the productive potential of the Park Nicollet Medical Center."[19]

"Although rapid change in a traditional profession is unsettling, we must avoid the temptation to try to slow things down and become spectators rather than participants," Nelson told the group. "We will be better served by anticipating change and providing leadership than by reaction to an environment where someone else is setting the rules."[20] While the new organizational dynamics created by joining the "two cultures" would take years to resolve, the leaders of the medical center had already turned to face the challenges of the market they were determined to help shape.

13

HARD LESSONS

PARK NICOLLET IN THE 1980S

By the time the Nicollet Clinic and St. Louis Park Medical Center merged in 1983, the Twin Cities health care market was well on the way to becoming a managed care market. HMOs enrolled 30 percent of the population and had begun to compete head on. Blue Cross Blue Shield and Physicians Health Plan (PHP) were enjoying tremendous success marketing their HMO products under the banner of "physician choice." The increased competition had introduced more insurance options, more attractive benefit packages, expensive advertising campaigns, and special services for the largest employers, but the escalation of medical costs continued unabated. Public concern over the costs of health care replaced access as the number one issue. Large Twin Cities companies, which had been "reticent to become aggressive, price sensitive purchasers of care," were now looking seriously at forming a "community buyers system" through which "HMOs and other insurers [would] be expected to bid for business."[21]

Health care had not escaped the national frenzy of consolidations, mergers, buyouts, and takeovers that overtook the economy in the 1980s. Nursing homes and hospitals were rapidly incorporated into national chains, creating a "dramatic shift in type of ownership and control . . . from non-profit to for-profit."[23] National HMOs were raising

Managed care refers to "any arrangement for health care in which someone is interposed between the patient and the physician with authority to place restraints on how and from whom the patient may obtain medical and health services and what services are to be provided in a given situation."[22]

capital and moving into new markets. Observing the scene in 1984, physician and editor of *Minnesota Medicine* Richard Reeves noted that "in 1983 alone, seven firms went public and brought in $280 million of private money—more than the [U.S.] government invested in seven years before it stopped subsidizing HMOs two and a half years ago."[24] This unprecedented influx of private money into health care, to the extent that it concentrated control of medical care into the hands of the insurance industry, was profoundly threatening to private practice physician groups, such as Park Nicollet, who had organized with the specific intent of retaining firm control over their workplace and the standards of medical practice.

As the pace of change accelerated, no predictions seemed too outlandish. HMO-guru Paul Ellwood, for instance, publicly expressed his view that health care in the near future would be dominated by only six to eight national management firms, or "supermeds," each commanding "revenues of $30 billion annually."[25] This scenario, while threatening to physician control of medicine, also promised vast opportunity for the more entrepreneurial leadership of MedCenters Health Plan and Park Nicollet. Might there not be room for a "supermed" designed and organized by physicians to serve the existing large multispecialty groups? These groups and smaller local clinics were scattered throughout the country and were only now experiencing the HMO revolution that had overtaken Minneapolis some ten years before.

AMERICAN MEDCENTERS, INC.

"Nelson saw a real market opportunity emerging, where we could work with other group practices and develop a plan and a long-term management contract with them," Loren

Vorlicky remembered. "We could then sell this concept of an HMO management company into the stock market, with the clinic owning the majority of it." A for-profit management company would create a conduit for private investment in the expansion of group practice HMOs, including MedCenters Health Plan, and allow for investing substantially in information systems, funding marketing efforts, and developing special benefit programs for large corporate clients. If the idea was successful, the clinic, as the majority owner, could expect a revenue stream independent of patient care that could fund the research and education aspects of the group's mission.[27] "Our competitiveness in Minneapolis," Glen Nelson recalled in 1995, "required an expansion of the capability of the HMO management, and expansion to other markets offered an opportunity to bring profits from those markets back into the Park Nicollet organization and add to the sophistication of the HMO management."[28]

"It was apparent that the physicians in PHP, for example . . . were losing control and were no longer able to set practice standards. My feeling was that if we could retain control of the financing organization, [group practice] had the capability to make the best medical decisions which would ultimately lead to real cost and market advantages."[26]

Glen Nelson, M.D.

As the idea of forming a for-profit management corporation developed in 1983, MedCenters Health Plan continued to flourish in the Twin Cities market. The plan added 27,000 new members, an increase which, in turn, contributed to the growing overload of patients in many departments at the clinic. The success of the health plan was pushing clinic facilities to the limit. "We didn't have the facilities, so . . . we couldn't take on more business," Stuart Hanson said, describing the board's discussion, "and [without more business] we didn't have any capacity to create the revenue to get the capital to build the buildings. It was a Catch-22. So somehow we had to get some capital, we thought, and this was the way." Park Nicollet and MedCenters Health Plan were not alone in choosing this course. Richard Reeves wrote in *Minnesota Medicine* at the time that "HMOs, profit or non-profit, need a surplus of money to grow. . . .This is why four of the largest non-profit HMOs—Group Health of Puget Sound, Group Health of St. Paul, Harvard Community Health Plan, and Health Insurance Plan of Greater New York—are forming a for-

The plan to create an HMO management company was not without precedent. The network started by Charles Bredesen and the Nicollet-Eitel Health Plan in 1981—three small HMOs in Eau Claire, Madison, and Neenah, Wisconsin—still existed in 1984. Managed by MedCenters, it had a combined enrolled membership of just over 20,000. The arrangement brought MedCenters increased visibility, a broader enrollment base to share administrative costs, and some recognition as a national HMO.[30]

profit corporation that would acquire and develop HMOs in regions other than where they operate."[29]

Although it was clear that the organization had very nearly reached the limit of its ability to borrow to support continued rapid growth, solid information on the developing financial crisis was months away. In late February 1984, after months of discussion and strategic planning sessions, the Park Nicollet Board approved the creation of American MedCenters, Inc., an HMO management company. The new company—led by Glen Nelson, David Jensen, and Loren Vorlicky—would use funds generated through stock sales to purchase the enrolled membership of MedCenters Health Plan, which would become the policy-making nonprofit sponsor of the health plan, as required under Minnesota law.

Contracting with MedCenters Health Plan

At the time of the creation of American MedCenters, no management company was concentrating efforts on the many group practices around the country who were "no longer sitting on the sidelines, but beginning to worry if they shouldn't get into prepayment themselves," as Loren Vorlicky put it in 1994. With an eye to developing this market, Glen Nelson had been working with a group of the largest western medical organizations on a business plan for a "national system of prepaid health care" that would be managed by American MedCenters. The American Federation of Clinics was interested enough to commit up to $60,000 toward the development of such a system in the spring of 1984.[31]

As American MedCenters was finalizing a management agreement with its home base, MedCenters Health Plan, Nelson returned from a meeting of the federation in Seattle with encouraging news. Of the twelve clinics who attended the July 5th meeting—clinics such as Scripps Medical Center, San Diego; Palo Alto Medical Center, Palo Alto;

the Mason Clinic, Seattle; and the Cleveland Clinic, Cleveland—eleven expressed interest in continuing discussions on the development of a national HMO network along the lines Park Nicollet/American MedCenters was proposing.[32] With the interest of these major players in hand, Nelson polled the physician staff of Park Nicollet in mid-July to gauge their reaction to American MedCenters, Inc., and no resistance was recorded. On July 23 the MedCenters Health Plan Board, still dominated by Park Nicollet physicians, voted to grant a contract to American MedCenters, Inc., for day-to-day operation of the plan beginning on October 15, 1984.[33]

AMERICAN MEDCENTERS, INC. FOUNDING BOARD, 1984

Glen D. Nelson, M.D., Chairman and CEO
David A. Jensen, President and COO
Loren N. Vorlicky, M.D., Vice Chairman and Medical Director
Charles C. Edwards, M.D., Scripps Clinic and Research Foundation
Donald L. Knutzen, General Mills
Richard L. Schall, Dayton Hudson Corporation

Establishing the New Company

Park Nicollet and MedCenters Health Plan worked together to put American MedCenters on a firm financial footing in preparation for its initial offering in the stock market. To accomplish this, American MedCenters purchased the assets of MedCenters Health Plan in October for $1.1 million in promissory notes. An additional $349,000 was promised to Park Nicollet for the purchase of the computer system that was then handling the information needs of both the clinic and the health plan. MedCenters Health Plan was granted an additional 160,188 shares of the new management company "in consideration for entering into the management agreement."[34]

Park Nicollet set up an endowment trust to hold its majority interest in American MedCenters. The board established the trust, corporate counsel David Lilly explained to the medical staff, to ensure that should the 3.1 million shares granted the clinic become valuable, they would not also "become the subject of covetous yearnings of individuals or small groups of our colleagues." Such a situation, he said, might "prove to be inimical to the social contract which underpins our operation."[35]

The founding trustees, named in October 1984, were Drs. Allan Kind and Earl Young, representing the clinic; L. S. DeSimone, then executive vice president of 3M, representing the Park Nicollet Medical Foundation; Glen Nelson, representing American MedCenters; and David Lebedoff, a University of Minnesota regent, representing "the public." The mission of the trust—to promote research and education, to maintain and improve the facilities of the clinic, to maintain competitive professional standards of compensation, and to maintain and improve the quality of medical care and support the practice of medicine at Park Nicollet—harked back to the mission statement established by the founding groups.[36]

Taking the advice of its financial consultants, American MedCenters granted its senior management—including clinic physicians Glen Nelson and Loren Vorlicky—substantial stock options in advance of the public offering. "We spent a huge amount of time internally trying to decide how we were going to live with that," Vorlicky said, "but it turns out you can't take a company public and expect to sell any stock unless the executives in the organization are incented to stay attentive to make it perform." The clinic board accepted this arrangement, although with some reservations.

Between July 1984 and the first sale of stock in January 1985, Nelson, Jensen, and Vorlicky worked feverishly to pull together the national group practice HMO concept, but by August it became clear that the politics and the scope of the project rendered it unworkable. Several of the major clinics involved—including Scripps Medical Center, the Mason Clinic, and the Cleveland Clinic—remained "interested in some type of working relationship with American MedCenters," Nelson told the Park Nicollet Board.[37] Ultimately, only the Mason Clinic entered into an HMO contract with American MedCenters. The contract, completed in 1985, created Virginia Mason MedCenters Health Plan, offering the services of the Virginia Mason Medical

Center, which included the Mason Clinic with 175 physicians in eight locations, the 312-bed Virginia Mason Hospital, and the Virginia Mason Research Center. The plan began operating in late December 1985.

Other efforts were more immediately successful. In December 1984, American MedCenters announced an HMO-development contract with the Fargo Clinic, a regional group practice with 125 physicians serving 140,000 people in eight cities. The new Fargo Clinic/MedCenters Health Plan, the first HMO in the Fargo area, was partially owned (20 percent) by American MedCenters. The Fargo Clinic was the primary provider and majority owner.

The Fargo HMO was fortuitously announced. The initial public offering of American MedCenters stock was made January 24, 1985, and the 1.4 million shares brought in more than $9 million. By April, American MedCenters became the sixty-sixth-largest publicly held company in Minnesota.[38]

With the infusion of capital from an enthusiastic Wall Street, American MedCenters HMOs continued to grow throughout 1985. Its "flagship plan," MedCenters Health Plan, became a regional presence. The addition of the Duluth Clinic, Ltd., the Interstate Medical Center in Red Wing, the Willmar Medical Center, and the Minnesota Health Network created a provider list of 1,219 physicians serving 212,700 plan members at 236 locations. In Georgia, American MedCenters entered into a joint venture with a physician group practicing with Atlanta Medical Associates. The resulting HMO, Georgia MedCenters, Inc., a hybrid of the group practice model HMO and the Independent Physicians Association (IPA), was designed as a prototype for areas of the country where there were few multispecialty practices. American MedCenters retained 51 percent ownership of this plan, and the 120-physician network began operating in February 1986. By the end of 1985, American MedCenters was managing seven HMOs covering more than 250,000 members and had increased net revenues by nearly 27 percent. Its stock price, however, had fallen from its initial high of $12.25 to between $8.50 and $6.25 in the fourth quarter of 1985, reflecting the market's disappointment that the major clinics had jumped off the American MedCenters bandwagon.

SHAKOPEE MEDICAL CENTER

In the sleepy town of Shakopee in 1972, four young general practitioners were ready to declare their independence from their older, more established partners. Medicine was moving forward. It was time to build, time to grow.

The four physicians—Donald Abrams, Joseph Keenan, Donald Lynch, and Anthony Spagnolo—formed a partnership and began making plans. With the support of the hospital administration and an influential local physician, Vror Pearson, the new group, Shakopee Medical Center, set up offices on the first floor of the St. Francis House next door to St. Francis Hospital in Shakopee. Less than a year later, in August 1973, the group moved into its new clinic building on East Tenth Street, designed by American Medical Building Guild of Madison, Wisconsin.

After moving into the new building, the group added Robert Christensen, a young general surgeon fresh from his Mayo residency. "We had made a conscious decision back then that our group would grow along the lines of a multispecialty group," Abrams explained. At the same time, David Fleming was hired as clinic administrator, and he became a full partner in the group in 1975. Two years later, the Shakopee group became a primary care provider for Medcenter Health Plan.

With the health plan behind them, the Shakopee group began to grow quickly. In late 1979 the group approved construction of a satellite clinic in the nearby community of Prior Lake, an option they had been considering since early

1975. "It was a smaller office designed for three physicians at one time," Abrams said, "and it was risky because as a rule of thumb you usually lose money in the first year or two with a new satellite." But the arguments for going ahead were compelling and by the time Abrams and Fleming were through "we'd outlined it right down to the last detail. . . . And it worked. . . . [When it opened] in 1981, not only did it not detract from our Shakopee base, the mother house, but it actually turned a profit all on its own," remembered Abrams. With this record, Fleming and Abrams became an attraction on the educational programs of the Medical Group Managers Association, lecturing on the process of constructing successful satellite clinics.

The group's referral relationships with St. Louis Park Medical Center were formalized in 1981 when regular hours were established for specialists to see patients at the two Shakopee facilities. With the economics of health care changing rapidly, the newly formed Park Nicollet, represented by William Costello, and the Shakopee Medical Center began serious merger discussions in 1984. For Abrams the decision boiled down to two things: Where do we fit best? Where are we going to fit in the future? "The key elements were the fact that Park Nicollet was a physician-directed clinic. . . . The president was a physician, the chief operating officer was a physician, and so forth, and we could relate to that . . . [and] they found us to be attractive I think because they knew us. They had done quality reviews through the health plan on a regular basis, so they knew what kind of practice we had." "It was our feeling," Glen Nelson wrote, "that integrating any group that was providing significant care for MedCenters Health Plan into Park Nicollet Medical Center offered opportunities for efficiency through common systems and improved quality."[39]

The nine family practitioners, two general surgeons, and fifty-two nurses and support staff of Shakopee Medical Center were welcomed into the Park Nicollet organization in

January 1985. Donald Abrams became the medical director of the southern region for Park Nicollet. His colleague Robert Christensen joined the Park Nicollet Medical Center Board and, coincidentally, was elected to chair the Board of Trustees of the Minnesota Medical Association that same year.

GOOD MEDICINE CONTINUES

Despite the whirlwind of stock offerings, mergers, and national strategies consuming the attention of top management, Park Nicollet continued to move forward largely unruffled. Guided by its ideals and mission, the organization continued to support efforts to examine and improve the quality of the medical care it provided.

Access

When the Quality Assurance Program revealed that nearly 30 percent of Park Nicollet patients consistently reported access problems, Diane A. Dahl, a family physician and Park Nicollet's first female board member, was tapped to chair the Task Force on Access to Care in 1983. Through the work of the task force, departments were urged to establish specific standards for access to care, to clearly define and communicate the availability of urgent care, and to actively recruit women physicians in response to "numerous patient requests."[40] Over the next eight years, Park Nicollet doubled its percentage of women on the professional staff from about 10 percent in 1984 to 22 percent in 1992 and increased the percentage of women physicians in the obstetrics and gynecology department from 25 percent in 1984 to 42 percent in 1992.

Prematurity Prevention Program

The obstetrics department during this period developed one of the first programs in the Twin Cities area to successfully reduce the incidence of prematurity and low-birth-weight babies. A collaboration with the perinatal program of Abbot Northwestern Hospital, the Prematurity Prevention Program was organized in 1984 by Leslie Pratt, an obstetrician who had joined St. Louis Park Medical Center in 1981. In less than one year the program had reduced the average hospital stay by one day. The program continued to reduce the number of newborns requiring intensive care throughout the decade, sparing untold trauma for newborns and new mothers alike and substantially reducing referral expenses for the medical center.[41]

Home Health Care Department

The home health care department was created in 1984 "to underscore the importance of patient and family education to promote a positive outcome."[42] Directed by Bonnie Roeder, a registered nurse, the department centralized management of various initiatives developed in the early 1980s to treat conditions at home rather than in the doctor's office or the hospital. These conditions included psoriasis, low back pain, wound treatment, and some intravenous therapies. The latter program alone saved 4,700 hospital days in 1984, worth more than $1 million.[43]

Senior Care Initiatives

In response to the growing numbers of elderly patients, Park Nicollet organized a division of geriatric medicine and health in 1984. The division was "formed to lead the development and direction of cost effective, coordinated programs for our elderly patients" and was committed to a "broad program of clinical care, health education, consultation, professional development, community service, and research."[44] One result was the creation of the patient education program "Over Fifty and Fit" in cooperation with the Park Nicollet Medical Foundation. The guided program of fitness, nutrition, and health information, under the direction of Gretchen Porter, R.N., and Stuart Hanson, received a national award of excellence from the U.S. Department of Health and Human Services in 1986.[45]

Technological Innovation

Despite tight finances, the group maintained their position at the head of the technological revolution in health care. The cardiology department developed a mobile echocardiography program to serve regional sites including Glencoe Hospital, Shakopee Medical Center, Methodist Hospital, and Fairview Ridges Hospital. A computerized tomography (CT) scanner was installed at Park Nicollet in 1984, and an agreement with Abbott Northwestern in 1985 allowed the Park Nicollet Radiology Department to become a principal user of the state's first fixed private magnetic resonance imager (MRI).

Children's Subspecialty Clinic

The pediatrics department, belatedly following the lead of its own Arnold S. Anderson, opened a new office in the Children's Medical Center complex in Minneapolis and later settled permanently in office space on East 26th Street. The new Children's Subspecialty Clinic was established in 1984 to provide convenient access to patients requiring intensive care at Minneapolis Children's Hospital. Ronald J. Glasser, a dual-certified subspecialist in pediatric nephrology and rheumatology who had joined St.

Louis Park Medical Center in 1979, and Steve Marker, a specialist in pediatric infectious diseases, who joined in 1980, organized the clinic.

CLINIC AND HEALTH PLAN GROW APART

The tremendous growth that characterized developments at Park Nicollet in the first half of the 1980s had all but overwhelmed the group's management systems by 1985. The 1983 merger had created a money-losing operation out of two groups accustomed to regular, if modest, profits. The deficit for 1983, reported in January 1984 to be a manageable $163,000, had grown to $242,000 by June and ballooned to a $2 million-audited-operating loss.[46] The clinic's financial performance in 1984 was equally dismal, with an operating loss of $2.9 million.

Why the medical center was suddenly and consistently losing money quickly became a contentious issue within the organization. James Stolhanske and Roger Upson, financial manager, were faced with a new, incompletely merged organization with two incompatible computer systems, a physician-compensation package that had been compromised upward during merger negotiations, rising wage scales for nurses and other personnel, and a heavy debt load at record interest rates on the new Burnsville and Brookdale satellites.

These internal issues were compounded by the shift in the group's medical practice away from hospital-based subspecialty care to the much-more-capital-intensive outpatient and primary care services required by their health plan patients. Shifting resources to primary care when resources were tight meant, among other things, losing the ability to pay competitive salaries for physicians in the hospital-based specialties. James Toscano—then the executive director of the Park Nicollet Medical Foundation, corporate secretary

"We ended up being in competition then with all these people in the community who also offered MedCenters Health Plan. I had patients leave my practice to go to Southdale Pediatrics under [the plan]. . . . We didn't feel MedCenters was particularly on our side anymore; they were on their own side."

Theresa Ryan, M.D.

for Park Nicollet, and a senior vice president at American MedCenters—said uncompetitive salaries led to shortages in departments like orthopedics. "We had a bottleneck . . . [in orthopedics which meant] we couldn't require everybody we were signing up to be part of MedCenters Health Plan to refer to Park Nicollet." This was translated by MedCenters/American MedCenters into an opportunity to increase patient choice in general. As a result, Upson told the board in August 1984, revenues from MedCenters Health Plan were $840,000 lower than planned for the first half of 1984. Decisions like this were good for MedCenters/American MedCenters and bad for Park Nicollet, Toscano reflected, and made it increasingly clear that their short-term interests were diverging.

With the inclusion of the Minnesota Health Network as a provider group in 1985, MedCenters Health Plan added primary care physicians in areas already served by Park Nicollet. "The expansion of the network," pediatrician Theresa Ryan remembered, "was always accompanied with the promise that, yes, you'll get more secondary and tertiary referrals." But that didn't help the primary care departments, who found themselves competing with other groups for MedCenters patients. Specialists at the clinic had their own complaints. Many had lost substantial portions of their referrals in the early 1980s when the Park Nicollet Board, in support of its exclusive relationship with MedCenters, chose to stay out of the Physicians Health Plan and Blue Cross Blue Shield AWARE preferred provider organizations. With a compensation system based largely on productivity, the financial consequences of the decision to exclude preferred-provider-organization patients were felt unevenly throughout the organization, creating a disunity unlike anything the organization had experienced. In spite of their technical ownership of the management company and control of the health plan board, the clinical group was becoming significantly alienated from both.

For their part, the physicians and managers closely associated with the health plan tended to believe that the clinic would weather the hard time if it could only adapt rapidly to the new realities of capitation. "They were great on the hospital side because they had good doctors . . . [but] they never engaged internal controls," said David Jensen. "They were still compensating doctors on a fee-for-service equivalency basis, which means everything was based on productivity, and you just can't function in a capitated environment on a productivity basis because it emphasizes procedures over medical intervention."

A health plan board member in 1984, Max Boller urged the clinic leadership to "assume the task of educating physicians on saving capitation dollars, for capitation is not at all clearly understood in the Medical Center."[47] The inability of the board to address this issue directly, according to Boller, "created a significant problem with physician morale." As the gap between the health plan's capitation payments and the clinic's fee schedule grew, a sense of antagonism developed between organizations that had every reason to work together.

Mario Petrini, who joined the Park Nicollet Board in 1985, agreed that the compensation system devised for the combined group was "schizophrenic," saying that "the more service we provided to patients, the more money the clinic lost; the better we got at utilization, the more the health plan cut our capitation; and, to make matters worse, the more each physician booked, the higher their individual salary." He added that the financial management systems in place at the time were also felt to be grossly inadequate to the task of managing a multispecialty group of more than 250 physicians. "When I came on the board, I was shocked at how little we knew about where the dollars were going," Petrini remembered. The clinic depended on generating new business and new prepaid contracts to support the discounted services it provided to MedCenters members. Market share was becoming increasingly expensive to capture and clinic facilities were nearing capacity. "It was rain-

"One of the things that I recognized was that whereas I went into this period right after the merger believing that the organization had many owners, I learned that there were actually a few owners, in terms of their willingness to put their shoulders to the wheel, and lots more customers."

Paul Batalden, M.D.

ing, but no one had their umbrellas up," is how Petrini summed up his sense of the organization in 1985.

Throughout 1985, the medical center board continued to back Glen Nelson and Paul Batalden, who had been named chief operating officer of Park Nicollet in 1985. In July, Nelson announced a "plan to balance revenues with expenses," a program he said would call for "the collective best efforts and teamwork among employees." A 5 percent hold-back on physician salaries was a central feature of the effort to cut expenses by some $2 million during the second half of the year. To the many physicians within the group who already felt underpaid, this was bitter medicine indeed.

With the storms of controversy swirling around the administrative suites, James Stolhanske decided to leave. Administrator since 1979, Stolhanske joined Beta Medical Management in Minneapolis for a brief time before moving to Florida to become the administrator for the Medical Center Clinic, P.A. At a board meeting in December 1985, Glen Nelson praised Stolhanske for his eighteen years of "loyalty and dedication to the medical center."

MCKINSEY REPORT

Painfully aware that recent events had "fragmented our shared values and defused our focus," Nelson agreed to hire outside consultants to assess the organizational structure.[48] McKinsey & Company, a nationally recognized business consulting firm, was hired to examine the business structures and relationships among Park Nicollet, Methodist Hospital, American MedCenters, and MedCenters Health Plan. In recognition of its growing stake in the success of Park Nicollet and MedCenters, Methodist Hospital agreed to split the cost of the project with Park Nicollet.

Beginning in September 1985, McKinsey interviewed key people in each of the organizations, conducted strategy sessions, and prepared financial and market analyses. The company's conclusions, reported at a board meeting in December, suggested that the interlocking leadership of Park Nicollet, American MedCenters, and MedCenters Health Plan was perceived as creating serious conflicts of interest and that this was at the heart of the growing conflict between the clinic and the health plan. The consultants went on to suggest, "To enable PNMC and AMED to pursue their separate interests without organizational disruption, an arms-length relationship between the two organizations should be established by physical and managerial separation. Leadership and management capabilities should be strengthened and a formal, working relationship between PNMC and Methodist Hospital should be established."[49] The tremendous growth of Park Nicollet and American MedCenters, they concluded, now required that each receive the attention of full-time management.

Max Boller remembers that a standing joke at board meetings in 1985 was about a farmer talking to a friend. The farmer says, "You know, I'm losing twenty-five dollars on every truckload of corn I bring in." His friend says, "Well, you're just going to have to drive faster."

The report was well received by the majority of Park Nicollet physicians and was roundly criticized by those people most closely associated with the health plan. Loren Vorlicky felt that McKinsey failed to recognize that "one of the really major strengths we had as a system was the overlapping leadership and interlocking board representation we had between the foundation, the clinic, and the health plan, able then to move all three organizations down the same path with an opportunity at least to integrate things." James Toscano, who had argued for a complete integration of the clinic and health plan in 1982, suggested that the report "reflected [McKinsey's] understanding of the traditional professional corporation. They did not yet understand the growing integration of the various elements of health care, what is now called managed care. They didn't understand what we were trying to do."

Moving down the same path, however, was no longer a high priority for the majority of physicians at Park Nicollet. Convinced of the need to pursue market dominance, the health plan, under the leadership of Nelson, Vorlicky, and

Jensen, had used Park Nicollet as the economic engine pushing the growth of MedCenters/American MedCenters, expecting that the long-term benefits of surviving as a major player in the HMO market would outweigh the short-term financial impact on the medical center. But the clinic was simply not strong enough in the Twin Cities market to sustain the strategy.

In an uncharacteristically terse annual report to the group, Nelson acknowledged that "1985 had proved in many ways to be the medical center's most challenging year of the past decade." The recommendations of the McKinsey consultants, he wrote, had "received broad (but not universal) acceptance." In order to implement the suggestions, he continued, "We will need new and additional leaders to direct us through a transitional health care environment. . . . It is essential that our systems and management be revised to meet today's needs, but such actions will be insufficient unless we draw together, focusing on our common purpose."[50]

After twelve years on the board and eleven years as president, Nelson bowed to the will of his colleagues and the McKinsey report and was succeeded by new leadership. Staying on out of loyalty to the group, Nelson devoted his energies full-time to American MedCenters as chairman during the transition. He then moved to an executive post at Medtronic, Inc. The new clinic board, which included four new members, elected James Reinertsen to serve as president and chair. It became his task to rebuild the group's confidence in their ability to move forward with a common purpose.

END OF AN ERA

True leadership is a risky business, with occasional misunderstanding and rejection the likely reward for tremendous vision and success in moving a group of people forward. In this light, the departure of Glen Nelson from clinic leadership in 1986 does little to dim his contribution to the group he led for eleven years.

Nelson succeeded Norman Sterrie in 1975 with a vision of building a multispecialty, private group practice of national significance. During his watch the group grew from 80 physicians to over 250 and enhanced their national reputation for excellence. A satellite clinic network was developed ten years before it became common practice. Membership in MedCenters Health Plan topped 200,000. A publicly traded HMO management company was launched. St. Louis Park Medical Center, the Nicollet Clinic, and Shakopee Medical Center had successfully merged. The International Diabetes Center was created. A major building was completed to meet the growing space demands of the constituent organizations. Park Nicollet's programs and innovations were copied in clinics around the country. The medical center and its associated organizations, under Glen Nelson's leadership, had become a mecca for the coming managed care revolution.

14

RESOLVING RELATIONSHIPS

PARK NICOLLET PREPARES FOR THE 1990S

JAMES REINERTSEN, NEW PRESIDENT AND CHIEF EXECUTIVE officer of Park Nicollet in 1986, found himself at the head of a group with deep reservations about their future. Rifts, factions, and operational problems remained from the merger of St. Louis Park Medical Center and the Nicollet Clinic; compensation was generally regarded as substandard; and the group had developed a deep distrust of their primary source of patients, MedCenters Health Plan. It was clear to Reinertsen that the fundamentals of group practice were sound but that "lack of management attention" and "a clumsy organizational structure" had "paralyzed decision making," "rotted away" the support staff infrastructure, and created "a physician group with poor morale, little cohesion, and an uncertain sense of ownership in the organization."[51]

Charismatic, articulate, and skilled at group process, Reinertsen was a natural choice to gather up the pieces of organizational unity and forge a new sense of shared purpose. With the board's approval, Reinertsen quickly brought in Joseph Mitlyng as chief operating officer to assist with the task. Mitlyng had spent ten years as associate director at the Marshfield Clinic and held a master of business administration degree from the Harvard School of

"McKinsey crystallized what we were against, but the first task I had was to create and build an organization around what we were for, not what we were against. We had to rediscover and rearticulate what we were, because this was really an identity issue."

James Reinertsen, M.D.

Business. Together Reinertsen and Mitlyng began to tackle the job of rebuilding the organization.

"One of the things Jim was fond of saying in '86," recalled Joe Mitlyng, "was that the clinic was experiencing a near-death experience. It helped, because it was pretty close to being accurate. The part of that statement that is really true is that what had happened before suddenly was of no consequence, because if we didn't figure out something pretty quick, we weren't going to have any money to pay staff. [With] turnover rates of 26 percent, and the bank wanting to call a $600,000 note, we weren't going anywhere."

THE "GET WELL PLAN"

The two new leaders immediately created what they called the "Get Well Plan," which outlined a package of financial and management changes designed to address the problems identified by McKinsey & Company in its 1985 report. The plan was presented to the staff in a series of meetings during the summer of 1986.

To implement the Get Well Plan, Reinertsen called on Donald Abrams, whose Shakopee clinic had merged with Park Nicollet one year earlier, to chair the McKinsey Steering Committee. The committee's job was to help reexamine and reshape the organization along the lines suggested by the McKinsey Report. Under Abrams' leadership, the committee established eight task forces to facilitate a ground-up review of the organizational structure and function in the following areas: values clarification, realignment with the health plan, hospital relations, the physician management structure, the role of the board, compensation, information systems, and administrative support. Reinertsen led the task forces on values clarification, realignment with the health plan, and hospital relations.

Other task force leaders were William Gamble (physician management structure), Max Boller (the role of the board), Rodney Dueck (compensation), and Joseph Mitlyng (information management and administrative support). Over a six-month period, the McKinsey implementation effort systematically drew all who were interested into a discussion of the future of Park Nicollet.

PARK NICOLLET MISSION STATEMENT, 1986

Our patients are our first priority. We have a strong sense of accountability to each other for providing outstanding care and service. We maintain our standards of excellence by active support of education, research, innovation, and professional growth for our entire staff. Furthermore, we reinforce our standards of practice by organizing as a physician-governed, professionally directed group practice. We serve the complete health care needs of the Twin Cities in an integrated system of care, and our many specialists also serve Minnesota and surrounding states. The mission of Park Nicollet Medical Center is to provide the highest quality health care and service possible.

Values Clarification

"I'll never forget those days," Reinertsen said of the values clarification process. "We spent five months on the subject with sixty, seventy, eighty people. . . . I said, 'Let's look back over our history and our actions and ask what they tell us about what we believe in.'" In the end, Reinertsen recounted, "We came up with a statement which not only defined our values, but in a sense also evolved a new definition of what our mission was." By fall 1986 the task force had boiled the core values of Park Nicollet down to one sentence: *Our patients are our first priority*. From that one sentence, a new mission statement was born.

Reinertsen sought and received assurance that the new statement embraced and communicated the founding values and ideals of St. Louis Park Medical Center and the Nicollet Clinic. Confident that the new leadership was on the right track, Reinertsen next launched "Patients First," an intensive staff education and dialogue process created to speed internalization of the values through all levels of the organization. Improving the clinic's relationship to its "first and most important asset"—the satisfied patient—not only would improve care, but also would go a long way toward ensuring the long-term loyalty of patients. "Patients First," Reinertsen wrote in 1987, "is designed to help us learn the skills to serve our patients better."[52]

Carol Hersman, a registered nurse who had joined St. Louis Park Medical Center in 1960, was director of patient care services in 1987. "The objective," she wrote about Patients First at the time, "is to improve the service orientation of our entire clinic by successfully managing our moments of truth."[53] Looking back on the initiative, she said, "People talked about Patients First for years afterwards. . . . We actually closed down clinics for half days so the whole staff could participate in the dialogue and presentations and so forth." At the very least, the program brought the clinic staff together to understand and work on the many challenges ahead.

Physician Management

The task force on physician management developed a plan to completely reorganize the group. "The Medical Staff Committee had more than twenty people, representing each of the subspecialties," Committee Chairman Gamble said. "It had become unwieldy and simply unable to reach a consensus on interdepartmental issues." The task force presented a streamlined organization chart that included a new Division Directors Committee made up of elected directors from each of seven medical divisions. The directors individually assumed management authority within their divisions and, as a group, assumed the policy-making role of the Medical Staff Committee. The medical director, who chaired the division directors meetings, reported directly to the president. Shortening the line of authority, the task force explained, "directs responsibility for decision making and accountability as close as possible to the individuals actually involved with the specific problems."[54] The board adopted these physician management changes in late 1986.

Information Management

The Information System Task Force examined the computer system and found an unstable combination of the various clinic and health plan systems operated by American MedCenters. The task force determined the combined system was too "fragile" to risk immediate separation. Mitlyng, however, began organizing an in-house computer department to regain control of Park Nicollet information systems at the earliest possible time.

In August 1987, Dennis Howard was hired to head the new information systems department. His first tasks were to install a new, dedicated IBM mainframe 3090 series computer and to manage the merging of three separate and incompatible scheduling and billing systems left over from the Nicollet Clinic, St. Louis Park Medical Center, and Shakopee Medical Center. By May 1988, five years to the month after the merger of St. Louis Park Medical Center and the Nicollet Clinic, a single IBM-based computer system was in place at all locations. The task of merging the three databases and purging the system of over sixty thousand duplicate records required thousands of hours of dedicated staff time and took the remainder of the year.

Most of the other task force initiatives were more complex and intertwined and required the patient perseverance of the administration and staff. In time, issues were unraveled, examined, and widely discussed, leading to many significant changes. The guiding principle, however, was a shared desire to refocus on the core business—providing medical care.

FINANCING THE SHORT TERM

The financial difficulties at Park Nicollet in the early 1980s were due in part to the group's efforts to maintain leadership in a rapidly changing health care environment, and part of this leadership involved being in the HMO business. The medical center had invested in establishing MedCenters Health Plan by agreeing early on to discounted fees and an end-of-the-month payment schedule. As

To combat the erosion of confidence in the leadership and to foster a sense of shared purpose, James Reinertsen and Joseph Mitlyng began "Third Thursday" briefings at which interested staff could hear the financial report firsthand and question the administration. This regular exposure to the financial end of the practice "changed the way we looked at our finances," according to Terry Ryan, who was then chair of the pediatrics department. "The physician staff would come to find out how the clinic was doing, and we began to feel more ownership for the problems."

the health plan grew, these arrangements created a tremendous cash-flow problem. With MedCenters now well established, Mitlyng and Reinertsen argued successfully in 1986 that payments should be moved to the beginning of the month. This small change, according to Joe Mitlyng, had a $4 million positive effect on the organization's month-to-month cash flow.[55, 56]

Real estate offered Park Nicollet administrators another opportunity to improve the financial picture. The transfer in 1976 of the St. Louis Park Medical Center buildings and grounds to the nonprofit St. Louis Park Medical Center Research Foundation created a stable and independent source of revenue to support research and education and also provided a more favorable tax situation for the then-profitable clinic. But by 1986 the separation of real estate equity from the main business of the group began to have a dramatic and negative effect on the group's debt-to-asset ratio—the amount the group owed versus what they owned. In the 1970s this was not an issue, because the amount of borrowing necessary was well within what the local banks were willing to finance based simply on the value of the group practice. But several years of million-dollar losses had driven long-term borrowing requirements beyond what the banks were willing to finance without collateral.

After analysis by Mitlyng and the board, negotiations with the foundation for the repurchase of the St. Louis Park properties began. At the same time, Mitlyng arranged to purchase the Burnsville and Blaisdell Avenue medical buildings, which were still owned by the Nicollet Clinic property company. "We were really desperate for assets," Mitlyng said, referring to the lack of collateral that was limiting the clinic's ability to borrow for expansion. But as much as the clinic may have wanted its central facility, the foundation was equally intent on preserving the long-term financial commitment to research and education, and the negotiations continued well into the 1990s.

SELLING AMERICAN MEDCENTERS

American MedCenters, Inc., the for-profit HMO management company organized by Park Nicollet in 1984, had by 1986 become a lightning rod for physician discontent. Under new leadership and facing another year of million-dollar deficits, the members of the Park Nicollet Board of Trustees, newly refocused on the group's core values, were ready to consider selling controlling interest in the company. "The group had declared, 'We are a multispecialty group practice,'" Reinertsen recalled, "'physician-governed, professionally managed, [and] committed to research and education. . . . We are a clinic. We are not a health plan. We are not a national HMO management company.'" This new focus was a big part of the decision to sell American MedCenters, Reinertsen said, adding "and we needed the money, and I honestly didn't think the stock was ever going to go anywhere."

Pediatrician Loren Vorlicky argued bitterly that the sale amounted to throwing away the dream of creating a unified health care system. He remains convinced that the decision to dismantle the overlapping relationships between the medical center, the foundation, and American MedCenters/MedCenters was rooted in the historic reluctance of physicians in group practice to "invest in what other industries would call the R&D side of their business." He later wrote that "the short-term financial gain was at the expense of long-term control over patient base, referrals and financial management."[57] William Telleen, Park Nicollet chief financial officer who arrived six months after the sale in 1986, agreed. "A major element of control was given up at that time," he said. "In hindsight, of course, the McKinsey recommendation to divest the HMO was not good advice. We are not now at the table when companies buy health insurance."

But whether another option existed in 1986 remains an open question. "Bringing MedCenters in-house at that point would have committed the group to an organization much like California's Kaiser Permanente," said Reinertsen, "and would have shut off referrals from the rest of the medical community." With many Park Nicollet specialists seeing more than half of their patients on a referral basis, this sort of integration would have "decimated the clinic as a specialty group and violated our sense of professional identity."

Future vision and strategy aside, the group had a major nonyielding asset in American MedCenters that, according to James Toscano, "had to be sacrificed to pay the bills. We wouldn't become the integrated managed care organization some of us wanted, but we needed the money to rebuild our basic organization."

Already looking for a partner that could provide the capital American MedCenters needed to finance an expansion into new markets, Glen Nelson adjusted his search to focus on potential buyers. By August 1986, Nelson and American MedCenters President David Jensen were negotiating with Partners Health Plans, a joint venture of AETNA Life Insurance Company and VHA Enterprises, a hospital management company. Negotiating for Partners was none other than Steve Goldstone, who had preceded Jensen in his former position as director of MedCenters Health Plan. The deal closed in September 1986 when Partners agreed to pay Park Nicollet $25.1 million for its 60 percent share of American MedCenters. The agreement laid out the payment schedule: $7 million in cash, a $9 million note, and another $9.1 million based in part on the growth of the plan.[58] American MedCenters continued operations as a wholly owned subsidiary of Partners Health Plans, and MedCenters, then the eleventh-largest HMO in the nation, became the largest HMO operated by Partners.

BREAKING WITH MEDCENTERS

The sale of American MedCenters gave Park Nicollet a little distance from which to examine and analyze its relationship with MedCenters Health Plan. From 1972 to 1986, the leaderships of the medical center and the plan were virtually indistinguishable. Always wary of outside forces gaining control of their professional practice, the physician-managers created an interlocking board structure to ensure the primacy of medical decision making and the medical group. This was effective in the 1970s, which were simpler times in the history of HMOs in the Twin Cities.

But by 1983 MedCenters Health Plan had grown into a powerful organization in its own right and was responding to the market according to its own interests, and the creation of American MedCenters in 1984 inserted accountability to public stockholders into what was becoming a stew of conflicting pressures. Within this context it is not surprising that the MedCenters board, still made up primarily of Park Nicollet physicians, saw growth of the health plan as the price that had to be paid for the long-term survival of both organizations.

The new Park Nicollet leadership lost patience with this strategy as the cost of treating MedCenters patients, more than 65 percent of the medical center's business, continued to rise faster than premiums. "Bill Telleen did a line of business analysis in the summer of 1987 that showed us we were losing $10 million a year on an operating cost basis," Joseph Mitlyng explained. "It was as if the [MedCenters] leadership had adopted a notion that somehow the health plan could succeed and the clinic could fail."

The immediate answer, Reinertsen and Mitlyng concluded, was to increase the percentage of fee-for-service patients seen at Park Nicollet, no small task in the health care market at that time. Fee-for-service insurance plans were shrinking rapidly as employees chose HMO and preferred provider plans. Blue Cross Blue Shield of Minnesota, once the standard of fee-for-service insurance, had exploded into the market with its own hybrid preferred provider plan called AWARE Gold which offered members both the broad choice of traditional indemnity insurance and the first-dollar coverage and no-paperwork advantages of the HMO.

Competing actively for the fee-for-service patient required two major initiatives. First, the identity of Park Nicollet needed to be separated from that of MedCenters. Market research done by Alan Dakay, Mitlyng's choice to head a new marketing department, showed that fewer than one out of four Minnesotans thought of Park Nicollet when asked to name a Minnesota medical facility. Sixty percent could not distinguish between Park Nicollet and MedCenters Health Plan, although eight out of ten recognized the name of the clinic when given a list of Minnesota institutions.[59] Adding fee-for-service patients meant creating a new public image. A TV and print media advertising campaign, "The other great clinic in Minnesota," was the first step.

Second, the exclusive relationship between Park Nicollet and MedCenters—which was a postmerger extension of the exclusive relationships both St. Louis Park Medical Center and the Nicollet Clinic had maintained with their respective plans—needed to be addressed. As David Jensen put it, "If there was a brand value to Park Nicollet, which I believe there was, that brand value was sustained by being exclusive." As late as the spring of 1986, Park Nicollet remained loyal by rejecting an attractive offer to participate in the AWARE Gold program. The Blues' interest in Park Nicollet, Reinertsen observed at the time, "was to use our participation to erode MedCenters Health Plan's solid foundation in the health care market."[60]

But as the interests of the health plan and Park Nicollet continued to diverge and net losses continued to mount on Park Nicollet's MedCenters business, AWARE Gold seemed to provide a viable solution. Consensus within the medical group began to move away from maintaining an exclusive relationship with MedCenters. "It would be easier for us to manage towards a goal of excellence in an environment where we participated in several health plans than to try to hide behind the marketing efforts of one plan," Reinertsen said in February 1987. "PNMC's long-term strategic position should be so good that health plans will compete for the right to use us."[61] To be "so good" required outcomes measurements that could be compared with those of other providers—a capability Park Nicollet could not develop on its own.

"AWARE Gold was a key part of this process," Mitlyng noted, "because we were able to negotiate a contract with the Blues, which provided 90 percent of our fees." In addition to a steady and growing stream of fee-for-service patients, the new relationship offered direct access to the Medisgroup outcomes data, a system that had just been installed in all metro hospitals by Blue Cross Blue Shield. The Medisgroup system—designed to provide comparative outcomes data—tracked key clinical findings to describe the severity of illness in patients who had different reasons for admission.[62] Blue Cross Blue Shield also promised up-front payment for medical research and patient education services to the cash-strapped clinic. "The money Blue Cross Blue Shield was able to put in at this point saved us," remembered Mario Petrini. Park Nicollet became a Blue Cross Blue Shield AWARE Gold provider for the first time in April 1987.[63]

Legal Challenges

Park Nicollet's decision was immediately challenged in court by the consumer members of the MedCenters Board, who were backed by the plan's new management company, Partners Health Plans. MedCenters contended that Park Nicollet's agreement with AWARE Gold violated their contract, which the health plan said excluded the clinic from a provider relationship with competing HMOs. This contention was soon rejected by the courts, thus legally freeing Park Nicollet from its exclusive ties to MedCenters; however, it brought into public view the increasingly strained relationship between the health plan and its founding group.

The familial bonds had been severed and the two organizations struggled to form a new relationship. However, MedCenters' lawsuit proved to be only the first spark of fireworks to come. After the lawsuit, Joe Mitlyng negotiated a provider contract with MedCenters that contained some assurances that Park Nicollet would not again be forced to accept capitation levels below cost. The contract also provided that the capitation levels would be set based on actuarial principles. As negotiations for 1988 approached, Mitlyng estimated that the clinic needed a 20 to 21 percent increase to return a 3 percent profit before risk.[64] This was rejected by MedCenters, which argued that its actuarial process supported a more gradual capitation increase of 11 percent in the first quarter with additional increases of 2 percent in subsequent quarters.[65] Under the new contract "we had the right to say whether or not we would take reimbursement below our costs," explained Joe Mitlyng. "If you think about it, it's the only way the relationship could work. Otherwise, you'd have a contract under which one party has all the power." Park Nicollet sued for arbitration.

After reviewing the data, the arbitration panel concluded that an 18 percent payment increase was reasonable. However, the Minnesota Department of Health, which was charged with regulating HMOs, decided to intervene at that point, citing concern that the increase might jeopardize the financial solvency of MedCenters. The department issued a cease and desist order prohibiting MedCenters from "implementing any portion of the January 21, 1988, arbitrator's award" or from "making any payments to PNMC which exceeded 1987 levels."[66] MedCenters, too, appealed the arbitrator's award based on the contention that its actuarial process was valid and that Park Nicollet's costs in several key categories were unreasonably high. After several years of court battles, the arbitration panel's jurisdiction was upheld by the Minnesota Supreme Court, but the dispute was not fully resolved until late summer 1990 when Park Nicollet agreed to give up its majority on the MedCenters Board, and the Department of Health agreed that the new formula for determining capitation levels was reasonable.

By the time of the annual meeting in early 1989, the clinic could celebrate a return to financial health. Describing the group's recovery, Mitlyng said, "In 1987, [the battleship PNMC] was low in the water, but in 1988 it was rising. Now after sixteen months of operating surpluses, our ship rides high and is regaining pride."[67] The Get Well Plan, along with good luck and good management, had succeeded.

CONTINUOUS QUALITY IMPROVEMENT

The goal Reinertsen had articulated, "to be so good that health plans will compete for the right to use us," had taken a more structured form by 1989. Under the guidance of Medical Director Rodney Dueck, the group began to invest in the concept of continuous quality improvement (CQI). Going beyond the quality assurance programs that had brought the organization national recognition, Dueck invited 3M quality management consultants to conduct a needs assessment to "serve as a baseline as we begin the quality management program."[68] Reinertsen and Dueck embraced continuous quality improvement as a philosophy of work uniquely suited to group practice medicine. The bottom-up emphasis helped to examine the process and not the people. This provided a structure for change in an environment where physicians and staff often reject changes imposed from above.

In fact, Paul Batalden and Loren Vorlicky had come into contact with Deming's ideas in the early 1980s and adapted them for the practice. Batalden recalled that he and Vorlicky found themselves in Atlanta, sitting in an auditorium with six hundred engineers listening to the eighty-year-old Deming talk about ball bearings. "The longer we sat in the course," Batalden said, "the more it seemed that he really wasn't talking about ball bearings. What he was talking about was a philosophy of work, the worker, the workplace, and the beneficiary of work. But the language of ball bearings would never do." Batalden translated Deming's ideas into words that would make more sense to doctors and nurses. Deming used the modified fourteen points in his book, *Out of the Crisis*. Deming's 14 Points Adapted for Medical Service are: [69]

1. Establish constancy of purpose toward service.
2. Adopt the new philosophy.
3. Require statistical evidence of quality of incoming materials.
4. Deal with vendors that can furnish statistical evidence of control. . . . Price of services has no meaning without adequate measure of quality.
5. Improve constantly and forever the system of production and service.
6. Restructure training.
7. Improve supervision.
8. Drive out fear.
9. Break down barriers between departments.
10. Eliminate work standards that set quotas.
11. Eliminate numerical goals, slogans, posters imploring people to do better.
12. Institute a massive training program in statistical techniques.
13. Institute a vigorous program for retraining people in new skills.
14. Create structure in top management that will push the above thirteen points.

Batalden tried unsuccessfully to get the clinic board to entertain Deming's ideas as early as 1982. Failing that and harboring a growing interest in continuous quality improvement, Batalden left the clinic to lead a group at the Hospital Corporation of America who were using Deming's ideas to create a model for health care. Dueck willingly concedes that Batalden was a key innovator in the field. "I think Paul was perceived as being brilliant, a broad reader, very articulate, and way ahead of his time," he said, even at the medical center which had a reputation around the country as being at the front edge of change. "But in Paul's world we were stick-in-the-muds."

Terry Shackelford was one of the first of a new generation of physicians specializing in general internal medicine at the clinic. He left the practice in the late 1970s and died of leukemia shortly thereafter. A group of physicians and the Shackelford family established an endowment in the foundation to fund a memorial lecture in his name. Held every fall, the Shackelford Lecture is the most important annual lecture at the clinic.

Dueck and Reinertsen continued to be interested in the management philosophy Batalden had begun to explore. For more than two years, the group's leadership studied Deming's management theories, visited other organizations who were using continuous quality improvement, attended seminars, and invited lecturers to speak on the topic. Dr. Donald Berwick, who headed quality control efforts at the Harvard Community Health Plan, dedicated his 1990 Terry Shackelford Memorial Lecture to the subject of quality. "In the end, he said, "complacency is the worst enemy of real quality. Beware the false logic of the old saying 'If it ain't broke don't fix it.'. . . If it ain't broke, it may just be that we don't know how much better it could be."[70]

To move continuous quality improvement forward in the clinic, Reinertsen and Dueck invited physicians to two half-day sessions on Deming's philosophy with the goal of producing quality improvement teams. "The reason Deming's theory of management has generated such excitement worldwide," Dueck wrote in 1992, "is that it offers a rational and effective method for not only improving and reducing cost, but also for rekindling the joy of our work."[71] Reinertsen wrote in his 1990 President's Report, "The CQI process is like the rudder on a boat—it helps us steer, to move efficiently, to avoid drifting in circles. We believe that Continuous Quality Improvement will eventually completely transform our clinic. This ongoing transformation is absolutely essential to achieving our challenging vision."[72]

The program developed rapidly, reaching into every aspect of the medical practice. Cross-functional teams were formed to refine administrative systems ranging from prescription refills to chemistry lab turnaround times, from forms management to contact lens remakes. Clinical teams

"I think things have generally gone very well. Park Nicollet has a national reputation for excellence, and is one of the largest clinics in the country. I feel very proud of what Park Nicollet represents now. I think it is a wonderful institution."

Robert Green, M.D., Founder

began working on the treatment of back pain, menopause, chest pain, urinary tract infections, breast mass, carpal tunnel, asthma, and many other conditions. The teams had at least three tasks, Dueck wrote in the *Bulletin*, "to work as a cross-functional team, to learn the theory and methods of CQI and to actually improve something."[73] Dueck and Reinertsen, taking to heart Deming's admonition that top leadership must be visibly committed to the process, personally facilitated several teams.

"The whole philosophy," Reinertsen said, "is very consistent with what the founders . . . believed in, that is to say, a data-driven approach to decision making, a scientific approach to medical care and its improvement, and a people-valuing professional approach to people management as opposed to an inspection and police-state kind of model."

Breast Mass Study

The success of the Breast Mass Study is one star example of the rapid and important change that the continuous quality improvement process made possible. The purpose of the study was to improve the process of diagnosing breast cancer. Publishing a report of this effort in the *Bulletin* in 1992, team leader and general surgeon Richard Migliori described how the paradigm helped to identify measurable quality indicators and the best current practices, as well as to develop a strategy for introducing the new process to the medical group at large.

"In any CQI process," Migliori said, "ideas for innovation and possible improvement come from listening to internal and external customers." For the Breast Mass Team, listening to patients revealed a willingness to consider almost any diagnostic option if it shortened the number of "sleepless nights." Listening to primary care physicians found them more than willing to relinquish diagnosis of suspected lesions to a radiological team. With these notable insights in hand, the Breast Mass CQI Team organized a radiological team to handle a new centralized diagnostic system and published a manual to share insights gained by the team.

Migliori cited his group's work as a good example of the important role of the Park Nicollet Medical Foundation in providing support for innovation and quality improvement work. "During the course of that team's work," Migliori said, "the foundation linked us with a benefactor who provided us with a stereostatic breast biopsy machine . . . and supported us in the process of doing a clinical trial comparing this new form of biopsy with conventional surgical biopsy." The results of the study reported a dramatic improvement in the process of care. "We were so enamored with it," Migliori remembered, "that we made it part of our standard process, a process [by which we can] now detect breast cancer a much higher percent of the time in its very early stages." The process also reduced the cost of the breast cancer detection biopsy from a high of $3,000 to well below $500. More importantly, it reduced the cycle time for the patient. Abnormal mammograms are now evaluated in less than three days rather than two to three weeks as before.

The continuous quality improvement program initiated by Reinertsen and Dueck continues to serve as the group's chosen strategy for maintaining Park Nicollet's reputation as one of the highest-quality health care providers in the state. As explained in the continuous quality improvement manual published in 1991, "Highest quality health service differs significantly from pure care. Whereas care is judged by professional standards, service is judged by whether or not we meet the expectations of our patients and other customers, such as referring physicians. *Care* is doctor knows best. *Service* is the customer is always right. . . . Our goal is to astonish our patients and referring physicians with excellent service."[74]

GOING NONPROFIT

The retirement of urologist David Anderson, a founder of St. Louis Park Medical Center, on December 31, 1986, marked a new milestone in the history of the medical group. For the first time since 1921, no founding members were practicing. The organization, which had prospered as a result of the ideals and hard work of the founders of the Nicollet Clinic and St. Louis Park Medical Center, had grown and matured into a beneficiary trust that was larger and more permanent than any individual. But despite its public commitment to education, research, and community service, the medical center was still organized and taxed as a for-profit corporation.

St. Louis Park Medical Center Administrator Roger Asplin had pointed out this anomaly in 1979 and recommended at the time that the medical group be merged with its nonprofit foundation. His research of what other large clinics in the Midwest were doing convinced him of the urgency of the project. The Internal Revenue Service, he reported, would continue to be skeptical of the close relationship between the nonprofit, tax-exempt research foundation and the for-profit medical center. Then President Glen Nelson accepted his reasoning and formed the Ad Hoc Organizational Options Committee consisting of Asplin, David Jensen, attorney D. James Nielsen, James Stolhanske, and James Toscano.

"The taxable nature of clinic earnings," Glen Nelson recalled, "favored a tax-averse strategy to dispense all income rather than build surpluses for investment." The proposed nonprofit status would have allowed for capital accumulation and, though there were no urgent financial problems, it was felt that the strategy had long-term advantages. To move the discussion forward, the clinic and the foundation formed a coordinating council in 1982 and charged it with organizing a thorough investigation of the proposed change. James Toscano was asked to chair the council and an implementation time line was established. Task forces on governance, professional development, and services presented a final report in August 1982, urging the group to formalize their role as a service organization dedicated to education and research. However, before the process could be completed, merger negotiations with the Nicollet Clinic and Nicollet-Eitel Health Plan became a higher priority.

"The reason the reorganization . . . didn't happen [in 1983]," explained Toscano, "is that we merged with Nicollet, and the lawyers said we had to wait a year for new financials . . . and by then something else had happened, and what had happened was American MedCenters." With the creation of American MedCenters and the worsening HMO price war, things got more complicated. Ultimately, the lack of revenue surpluses sapped the feeling of urgency from creating a nonprofit entity.[75]

By 1988 the urgency had returned. Park Nicollet was again beginning to generate surplus revenues, which were taxable. "As we got into 1988 and could see we were going to make money, then it became time to start worrying about the idea of tax-exempt status again," Mitlyng noted. With the help of Robert Bromberg, an attorney with Paxton and Seasongood of Cincinnati, the acknowledged authority on medical group practice tax issues, a proposal was prepared and put to a vote. In September 1988, the physician beneficiaries of the trust voted 138 to 2 in favor of seeking tax-exempt status. By September 1989 the Internal Revenue Service granted full tax-exempt status retroactive to 1985.[76] This ruling produced a tax savings of just over $3 million.[77]

The savings was important but, according to Reinertsen, "Perhaps an even more cogent reason was, somebody said, 'Look, we have been functioning as if we were a nonprofit . . . Why don't we get the tax credit for it?'" And there was another reason. "I was still quite fearful that the Philistines might come in and take over the values of the clinic at some time," said Reinertsen, "and I said, 'Isn't there a way that we could perpetuate the legacy of the founders of our clinic and make sure it would never change?'" The answer lay in the creation of a public foundation that "in effect made the promise to God, country, and the IRS, for time immemorial, that we would do the things the founders put us together to do."

PHYSICIAN COMPENSATION

Through all of its various iterations since 1921, Park Nicollet depended on the experience, training, and conservative practice styles of its physicians, and the atmosphere of a collegial group to ensure a consistently high standard of care. Committed as well to the traditions of fee-for-service private practice, the group calculated physician compensation largely on the extent of individual bookings. As Max Boller put it, "The physicians, even in St. Louis Park, were always leery of socialized medicine, staff model HMOs, the British system," and by and large resisted attempts "to tinker with the fee-for-service system."

Over the years, however, the economics of group practice changed along with the medical marketplace. The growth of MedCenters had turned traditional ideas of productivity upside down. "The clinic's interest to conserve resources through reduced utilization," Mario Petrini said, "was in conflict with the personal incentive to generate bookings." Failing to adjust incentive systems to reflect the changed environment, Petrini said, was one of the reasons the group was in such a deep financial hole by 1986. Over the next five years, primarily through the leadership of Charles Jacobson in helping the group to better understand managed care, physician income was largely disconnected from procedures performed.

The obstetrics and gynecology department was the first to take steps in this direction in 1988. A new formula called for 80 percent of the department's total compensation budget to be distributed on an equal basis, and the remaining 20 percent was to be allocated based on a combination of productivity and longevity. William Gamble remembered that de-emphasizing productivity, "encouraged us to practice as group and not as individuals. For example, to encourage physicians to refer patients with subspecialty surgical problems to the person in the department who had the most experience and expertise in dealing with that particular problem, as opposed to doing it yourself in order to generate a bookings value and therefore income." Migliori added that ". . . we wanted physicians to worry more about the processes of care rather than the processes of generating an income." Over the next several years all departments made the switch to straight salaries for physicians, with a small incentive package for longevity, productivity, and academic or administrative effort.

STRENGTHENING TIES TO METHODIST HOSPITAL

Methodist Hospital was also in transition. With a proud tradition of quality care and an enviable position as the lowest-cost hospital in the region, Methodist Hospital had remained robustly solvent. Administrator Earl Dresser, nearing retirement age, was planning for the future and looking for ways to ensure the future of his hospital in the new era of consolidation and competition for the health care dollar. Low-profile negotiations with Park Nicollet and others "to create a horizontally and vertically integrated system" were underway as early as 1984.[78] Although these talks foundered, the exploration served to highlight the interdependence of the two organizations. With more than 30 percent of its patients coming from Park Nicollet and MedCenters Health Plan, Methodist had a keen interest in maintaining the close ties established with the clinic when the hospital moved to St. Louis Park in 1959.[79]

For its part, Park Nicollet had an opportunity to translate this interdependence into an additional measure of financial support. The low-cost position of Methodist, Reinertsen told Terry Finzen, Earl Dresser's successor, was due in large part to the practice methods of Park Nicollet physicians. The hospital had been able to remain independent through the first wave of hospital consolidations—kept busy by the network of primary care offices, by MedCenters, and by the efforts of Park Nicollet physicians who had set up many of the specialty centers at the hospital. Ensuring the short-term economic health of Park Nicollet, Reinertsen argued, was simply good business for the hospital.

Reinertsen's arguments impressed the hospital board. By January 1987, an agreement was signed between Park Nicollet and Methodist Hospital, outlining areas of expanded cooperation in return for a one-time payment of $2.5 million by the hospital to Park Nicollet. "The basic idea," Mitlyng said, "was to get a discount on the price that we were paying [for hospital services] beyond what they had been giving us before." In return, he said, "we would continue to do some things, continue to use them for CT and MRI services, for example." The agreement provided a financial boost for Park Nicollet at a critical time.

TOWARD AN INTEGRATED CARE SYSTEM

While the agreements of 1987 created a better understanding of mutual interests between Park Nicollet and Methodist Hospital, it became clear by 1989 that the two organizations were still working at cross-purposes and unable to economically develop joint venture projects.

"The hospital really was piece by piece trying to build a clinic of its own by putting together associates, supporting independent physician practices, and putting together outpatient facilities and services," Reinertsen said, and "the clinic was going about building the bits and pieces of a hospital. . . . We were doing things that I would regard as somewhat unseemly for nonprofit community resource organizations to be doing, not dissimilar to what was going on around the rest of the country by the way. . . . But nevertheless, we were bothered by it in the sense that it was inconsistent with our mission to be putting money into these kinds of duplicative resources for the community that simply added cost."

A massive consolidation among hospitals in the Twin Cities was also putting pressure on Methodist to secure its market share, now more than 60 percent dependent on Park Nicollet. No less than ten Twin Cities acute care hospitals were closed between 1986 and 1993.[80] On the other side, Park Nicollet was struggling to find the resources it needed to keep abreast of the latest technology and ahead of the demand for its services. Still, there was resistance within both organizations to integrating further.

Reinertsen and Mitlyng proceeded carefully in negotiations with Terry Finzen and Robert Galloway, president and chief executive officer of Methodist. Affiliation talks began in earnest late in 1989. The details were hammered out at meetings that continued throughout 1990 and most of 1991. The resulting agreement, initialed by Reinertsen and Galloway on December 11, 1991, created the framework for the "first private, integrated health care system of this type and size in the Minneapolis area."[81, 82]

Reflecting the caution on all sides, the affiliation agreement created a parent board that would coordinate the integration of care. The existing Park Nicollet and Methodist Hospital boards would retain title to their property and continue to elect their own chief executive officers. "It was really a cumbersome model," Reinertsen admitted. "It was not really integrated management and governance, but it was what was politically feasible."

With the lessons of the 1983 merger fresh in their institutional memory, the group felt in no mood to rush into a shotgun marriage. So what resulted, Reinertsen explained, was "an engagement agreement. It said we promised to get married by the end of 1993 if we could plan the wedding without blowing apart." Don Amren, vice president of medical affairs at Methodist Hospital in 1995 and a pediatrician at Park Nicollet since 1963, suggested that the engagement was long overdue. "Many of us who had been at the medical center for a long period of time felt the movement toward getting together was a natural thing that should have occurred ten to fifteen years earlier."

After more than thirty years of sometimes difficult collaboration, the two organizations had taken a large step toward a more complete integration of patient care services. In an era characterized by uncertainty and change, Park Nicollet and Methodist Hospital had each chosen a care partner they knew well.

15

FACING THE FUTURE
HEALTHSYSTEM MINNESOTA

THE CREATIVE TENSION THAT CHARACTERIZED THE RELATIONSHIP between Park Nicollet and Methodist Hospital carried over into their new affiliation. Carefully crafted to preserve the independence of two equal partners, the agreement signed in December 1991 set clear boundaries for the parent organization temporarily called "NewCo." Its objectives were to create a system of cooperative planning, to develop a vision for an integrated health care organization, and to generate immediate administrative cost savings. However, during the "engagement" period, both sides retained an ultimate veto over all organizational and management proposals.

The agreement created the Joint Committee of the Boards to steer the transition. Robert Galloway, president and chief executive officer of Methodist Healthcare, Methodist Hospital's parent company, and James Reinertsen, president and chief executive officer of Park Nicollet, co-led the joint board committee. The committee created five task forces to address compensation and benefits, operating principles, a facility plan for the main campus, a facility plan for remote campuses, and a quality plan. A new mission statement declared that the combined organization would strive "to be the premier comprehensive regional health care system in the nation."[83] In August 1992

JOINT COMMITTEE OF THE BOARDS
JANUARY 1, 1992[84]

Don Amren, M.D.
Rodney Dueck, M.D.
Terry Finzen
Robert Galloway
John Herman
Charles Jacobson, M.D.
Joseph Mitlyng
John Reichert, M.D.
James Reinertsen, M.D.
William Shimp, M.D.

"We gave ourselves plenty of opportunities to say no, but it seemed to be the right idea, so we came together in 1993, not as a hospital acquiring a clinic, not as a clinic acquiring a hospital, but as a very even, 50/50 kind of deal."

James Reinertsen, M.D.

the joint committee chose Galloway and Reinertsen to be co-presidents of the organization, with the titles chief administrative officer and chief quality officer respectively.

Reinertsen and Galloway methodically moved the planning process forward. Within months, it became clear that the organizational structure was unnecessarily complicated and unwieldy. "Nobody would argue, even at the time, that it was the best possible structure," Reinertsen said. "It had two presidents and a relatively cumbersome board structure. Each of the subsidiaries had their own board, and the CEOs of the subsidiaries . . . reported to the subsidiary boards, and only in a murky way to the presidents of the system and the system board. In other words, it was a little loose, although, again, highly typical of integrated care system models around the country." In June 1993 the new organization was named HealthSystem Minnesota: The Healthcare Network and became the parent company of Park Nicollet, Methodist Hospital, Methodist Hospital Foundation (a subsidiary of the hospital), and Methodist Associates, which owned the Methodist properties.[85]

HEALTHSYSTEM MINNESOTA BOARD, JUNE 2, 1993

OFFICERS

Robert L. Galloway,
President and Chief Administrative Officer
James L. Reinertsen,
President and Chief Quality Officer
Geoffrey L. Kaufmann,
Vice President, Strategic Planning and Corporate Development

(continued)

BUSINESS HEALTH CARE ACTION GROUP

In the 1990s, health care reform was again set to resume its position at the head of the national agenda. The Minnesota legislature considered a universal health care proposal called HealthSpan in 1989, which was backed by a coalition of citizen groups and providers. Although the bill failed to win much support in the health care industry and subsequently failed in the legislature, HealthSpan helped focus the attention of the "Great State of Health" on the state of its health care system.[86]

The transformation of medicine in the Twin Cities was proceeding rapidly. In 1991, the same year that Park

Nicollet and Methodist Hospital announced their affiliation agreement, Physicians Health Plan and the SHARE Health Plan merged to create Medica, one of the largest HMOs in the country with 540,000 members.[87] Group Health and MedCenters were talking of forming a partnership with sufficient geographic breadth and financial depth to challenge Medica and Blue Cross Blue Shield.

At the same time, Twin Cities employers were understandably frustrated with the continued escalation in the cost of employee health care benefits. Although costs in the Twin Cities were some 20 percent lower than the national average, the rate of growth was 12 to 15 percent, four times the rate of inflation.[88] A handful of major employers began to organize a new coalition to pool their purchasing power. The Business Health Care Action Group, or "BHCAG" as it soon became known, began operating as a buyers coalition in the fall of 1991. Its fourteen original members, with fifty thousand employees in the Twin Cities, included many of the same companies that had actively supported the HMO movement in the early 1970s. General Mills and Dayton Hudson, for instance, both key members of BHCAG, had been members of the earlier Twin Cities Health Care Development Project and before that had supported St. Louis Park Medical Center in its formative years. Together, BHCAG companies were spending some $200 million on health care each year, 6 percent of the Twin Cities market.

As president of the SHAPE Executive Fitness Program, Reinertsen was in close contact with many Twin Cities CEOs and health benefits administrators. "Here was this business group that we had been talking to behind the scenes for some years," Reinertsen said. "We had been asking, 'Why don't you buy based on documented quality and cost? Why don't you buy from organizations that can do things in a consistent way?'" The business community's answer to these questions was put together by BHCAG in early 1992 in the form of a request for proposals (RFP),

Board of Directors

David D. Koentopf,
Chair, Everest Medical
Donald E. Benson,
Vice Chair, MEI Diversified
Stanley R. Nelson,
Vice Chair
Dee Kemnitz,
Secretary, Carlson Company
Carl R. Pohlad,
Treasurer, Marquette Bancshares
Gail P. Bender, M.D.
Douglas R. Coleman Jr.,
Dain Bosworth
Terry S. Finzen,
Methodist Hospital
Donald W. Golfus,
Apogee Enterprises
Charles L. Jacobson, M.D.,
Park Nicollet
Richard H. King
Kermit B. Knudsen, M.D.,
Scott and White Clinic, Temple, Texas
Wayne F. Leebaw, M.D.,
Endocrinology Clinic of Minneapolis
Kenneth A. Macke,
Dayton Hudson
Richard J. Migliori, M.D.,
Park Nicollet
Lewis M. Mithun,
R.O.M. Financial Services
Joseph W. Mitlyng Jr.,
Park Nicollet
John E. Pearson,
Northwestern National Life Companies
William F. Schoenwetter, M.D.,
Park Nicollet
Arthur R. Schulze

which asked providers to submit bids for BHCAG's Employee health care business.

To win the contract, BHCAG told its potential applicants, a provider needed to demonstrate a commitment to deliver high-quality, cost-effective care; to eliminate unnecessary and inappropriate care; to objectively document a continuous improvement in health-care service delivery and outcomes; to offer an integrated system of care that would emphasize continuity and coordination; and to manage the totality of care required by employees and their families.[89] In return, BCHAG would handle all administration and reimburse providers on a modified fee-for-service basis. "This RFP was a fifty-mile-an-hour fastball down the center of the plate," Reinertsen said. "It was exactly tailored to what we could do. The trouble was [we] couldn't serve all of their employees."

The solution to this dilemma was already in the works. In January 1992 a joint committee of the boards of MedCenters and Group Health began discussions to form what would later that year become HealthPartners. The resulting agreement was announced in April 1992, an event William Schoenwetter, then a director of MedCenters, termed the "most dramatic step MedCenters has taken in its twenty-year history," which "represents a milestone in managed care development."[90]

GROUPCARE CONSORTIUM

Reinertsen remembers putting in a phone call to George Halvorson, then president and chief executive officer of Group Health. "I called George and said, 'Why don't we create, for purposes of this bid, the functional equivalent of an integrated care system across our boundaries. We won't merge the doctors, but we'll get them working together as professionals, so we can deliver what BHCAG is asking for.'" Halvorson was enthusiastic and soon an outline of the resulting GroupCare Consortium was being sketched by Halvorson; Reinertsen; Kirby Erickson, chief executive officer of MedCenters; Dr. Paul Brat, medical director of Group Health; and Joseph Mitlyng, chief operating officer of Park Nicollet.

By all accounts BHCAG was interested in more than "trying to bargain for better rates; they [were] also trying to apply the industrial principle of continuous quality improvement to what they perceive[d] to be a splintered, complex, overutilized and costly system."[91] "We needed to promise BHCAG," Reinertsen explained, "that if a patient came into an office of a doctor in Woodbury that they'd get the same care process as if they came to a doctor in Maple Grove, and we had no way of doing that short of working together professionally."

As the GroupCare proposal came together, it fell to Rodney Dueck, Park Nicollet's medical director, to turn the clinic's experience in continuous quality improvement and outcomes management into an operational plan acceptable to the BHCAG reviewers. "I was given this book on a Thursday, the BHCAG RFP," Dueck remembered, "and they said, 'We want you to provide all the information on quality, and we want it on Monday.' I was planning to leave on a vacation to take my son to visit colleges, and so for the entire trip I sat in the back seat of the car and dictated seventy pages of detailed responses to all these questions they had." The only reason it was possible to complete the assignment at all, he noted, is that "their RFP was our strategic plan." Having spent several years working through the implementation of a Deming-style management plan was a tremendous advantage, Dueck said. "Our competitors simply had no idea what [BHCAG was] looking for."

Reinertsen led the development of the integrated quality improvement program Dueck had outlined. The result was an agreement in July 1992 to fund a new joint clinical guidelines institute, the Institute for Clinical Systems Integration (ICSI). Reinertsen, who left his position as chief executive officer of Park Nicollet in August 1992 to become president and chief quality officer of HealthSystem Minnesota, was tapped to lead ICSI. Charles Jacobson, an endocrinologist and Park Nicollet board member who had pioneered efforts to understand issues of physician utilization in a capitated environment, was elected to replace Reinertsen as president and chief executive officer.

In less than five months, the GroupCare team had put together a cooperative network of the region's largest medical groups that "would transform how we diagnose and treat illness," as Paul Brat told the *Star Tribune*. The effort was rewarded in July 1992 when BHCAG awarded a three-year contract to GroupCare Consortium. Dr. Bryan Bushick, a BHCAG consultant, said that the key factor in the decision was that GroupCare was the only health care system that had already instituted programs to control cost and quality.[92] According to Steve Wetzell, executive director of BHCAG, GroupCare won the bid "because there was more potential for provider empowerment and involvement in the way their bid was structured."

The success of the GroupCare proposal sent a powerful signal to the Twin Cities health care market. Gordon Sprenger, chief executive officer of HealthSpan, told the *Wall Street Journal*, "Our challenge is to give up some of our individual autonomy to provide the kind of disciplined product that GroupCare provides." The name of the consortium was changed to HealthPartners in August 1992 after Group Health and MedCenters Health Plan merged, and HealthPartners became the primary insurance carrier for BHCAG. George Halvorson was named president and chief executive officer of HealthPartners.

INSTITUTE FOR CLINICAL SYSTEMS INTEGRATION

Within the GroupCare partnership, the Institute for Clinical Systems Integration was responsible for the development of clinical guidelines. Over the next three years ICSI developed into a tripartite organization, forming divisions to examine the population's current health status and needs; to provide statistical analysis of the outcomes of treatment; and to develop guidelines for current best processes.

The unique element in the GroupCare proposal, Steve Wetzell said, was ICSI. "There was no other bid that came up with that kind of innovative approach to engage the providers in process reengineering. Bringing ICSI into the market through the way we wrote that proposal in 1992," Wetzell continued, "has been one of the two most meaningful accomplishments" BHCAG can claim in the Twin Cities market. "It's actually pretty remarkable what the medical groups have done through ICSI, because the (financial) incentives actually work directly against the work that is being conducted through the Institute," Wetzell said in late 1995.[93]

While it can be difficult to find enough common ground among physicians to write a guideline on a given subject, implementation in day-to-day practice is universally regarded as the greatest challenge. Surgeon William Gamble agreed that implementation "is still a big stumbling block. You can create a critical pathway, but unless you have some way of building automatic implementation into the system, doctors have difficulty in getting rid of old habits."

It is a fact, Dueck acknowledged, that the ICSI guidelines have not been uniformly implemented. But the failures have been instructive, and the positive results achieved through the guidelines prove their value. "Deming told us that unintended variation is a source of waste," Dueck said,

"We are regarded nationally as being on the front edge of the push to implement guidelines. Systems around the country come here and interview with us about how we do it. When they come, we tell them all our faults and all of the places we've screwed up. One comment we got back from Henry Ford Medical Center was 'Your success is exceeded only by your self-criticism,' which I think does reflect some of our culture."

Rodney Dueck, M.D.

referring to the quality improvement teacher W. Edwards Deming. "What we found, when we started to look, is that there is enormous variation in the care that is provided. For example, for urinary tract infections, UTIs, we found that if a patient would pick up the phone and call one doctor it would cost them $6 to get their UTI problem solved and, if they ended up with another doctor, within the same organization, it would cost them $139. . . . Well, a guideline is simply the result of having a group of people who are given the time to study the medical literature, study current practices, study the results, and ask, 'What is the best process?'—not the cheapest—'What is the best process?' It just turns out that the best process typically costs less." After the guideline for UTIs was implemented, he noted, the average cost dropped from $60 to $20.

"These are living guidelines," Richard Migliori explained. "Our physicians have the privilege of not using them, provided they are willing to share with us the reason why they've deviated. In the majority of cases, they do it for a very good reason. Then we look at why, and, if it happens frequently enough, then we change the guidelines."

FACING THE FUTURE

As chief quality officer, Reinertsen argued forcefully that to meet its stated goals and flourish in the new health care marketplace, HealthSystem Minnesota (HSM) would have to increase its "systemness." In his first annual report to the board, Reinertsen lauded the "remarkable degree of collaboration and cooperation" that had occurred during the first ten months of operation, in spite of a cumbersome structure that provided "too many opportunities for us to make decisions which are in the best interests of each compartment of HSM but not in the best interest of HSM as a whole."[94]

Pressure was building at Park Nicollet to take the merger to the next level. After a few years of steadily rising premiums, the health care market was tightening again. Efforts to reduce the unnecessary utilization of services were creating mixed financial results—increasing HMO revenues but decreasing fee-for-service income at a time when fee-for-service patients were a growing percentage of the clinic's business. A worried chief financial officer, William Telleen, pointed out in late 1993 that the guidelines were improving the financial results of serving prepaid HMO patients, but worsening the results of the same service to fee-for-service patients, including most Medicare patients. The solution was to enroll more HMO patients without adding clinical staff. But the HMO enrollment increases projected for 1994 failed to materialize, due in part to patients switching from MedCenters to BHCAG and the abandonment of HMOs by the small-to-midsized employer groups.

"The large employers and policy wonks appreciate HSM because of the 'only' aspects of our system," Reinertsen said in 1993, noting the ability of the system to dramatically reduce utilization of physician services through innovations such as the ICSI guidelines and nurse phone-care services. "But patients and their families (and a substantial portion of our reimbursement system)," he went on, "are still focused principally on the 'all.'" Patients and the smaller employers, he said, were not choosing providers based on the ability to deliver consistently outstanding care, but on relationships, service, and price. "Our challenge is to stay in business and to grow, even though our current consumer and reimbursement environment isn't entirely congruent with our aim."[95]

The success of the reorganization efforts, Reinertsen commented, would be "vitally dependent on whether or not the resulting structure has enough central nervous system and backbone to make and implement the tough decisions necessary to improve the performance of HSM as a system." If HSM is to realize its full potential, he concluded, "it will have to have the courage to become a 'system' in the true sense of the word. Not a collection of semiautonomous organizations. Not a gaggle of frightened organizations huddled together for defensive purposes. HSM must become a system in which all our processes and people work cooperatively together to achieve our aim."[96]

Frederick Engstrom, then chair of the mental health department at Park Nicollet and a member of the HealthSystem Minnesota Organization Committee, said that in struggling to rationalize the executive compensation structure, the committee soon understood "that by having two separate organizations, even though we had a promise to do joint planning, each organization was still benefiting at the expense of the other. We realized, for instance, that executives at Methodist were getting big bonuses based on meeting annual targets which they could meet by beating out Park Nicollet. The [Organization] Committee, which was mainly community members like Dave Koentopf and Art Schulze, realized that, if we were going to merge, then we really had to have an asset merger and really have one system rather than two parallel systems."

With that understanding, the Organization Committee moved ahead in the spring of 1994 to choose a new chief executive officer. Three finalists were interviewed extensively, including James Reinertsen; David Koentopf, first chair of the HealthSystem Minnesota Board; and Charles Jacobson. Robert Galloway had taken himself out of consideration earlier, announcing that he would retire that summer. It was at this point, Engstrom noted, that the tension began to build. At stake was not only who was going to be the new chief executive officer but also, more importantly to Park Nicollet, what sort of governance would be adopted. Abandoning the semiautonomous structures meant, above all, abandoning what little remained of the long tradition of physician ownership of the group.

Very early in the process, Jacobson, in a report to the Park Nicollet Board, spelled out a list of fifteen principles by which the reorganization should be guided. First on his list was "physician leadership - professional management."[97] So, when the committee began meeting in March 1994, Engstrom said, he and Richard Migliori, the two Park Nicollet representatives, "really had two agendas. One was to choose the CEO and the other was to lay the groundwork for a true merger. So Dick Migliori and I kept pushing and saying we had to do both agendas," Engstrom continued. The result was a two-part process: first, agreement on general principles; second, detailed changes in the bylaws. All three boards—Park Nicollet, Methodist Hospital, and HealthSystem Minnesota—then had to sign off on each step.

Ultimately, Engstrom remembered, it was Dick Migliori who "really very eloquently convinced the others that Reinertsen had not only the personal qualifications, but that he had shown an ability to bring us out of a state of near bankruptcy, and had shown an ability to be really tough with the medical staff on important issues." By late June, the committee had completed both parts of its agenda. It had nominated Reinertsen for chief executive officer, and it had outlined a structure and a set of organizing principles that Migliori and Engstrom felt would be acceptable to Park Nicollet physicians. The most important of these provisions allowed for an elected Park Nicollet Management Committee to nominate a majority of members to any future chief-executive-officer evaluation and nomination committees and to veto any future changes in the bylaws of HealthSystem Minnesota.

Still, it was not an easy decision for the Park Nicollet Board. "The night before the vote," Engstrom said, "we argued late into the night and finally disbanded without being sure how we would vote the next day." Ultimately, however, all three boards approved the plan for a complete asset merger and chose James L. Reinertsen as president and chief executive officer of HealthSystem Minnesota. After a few more months of work, the bylaws changes needed to complete the HealthSystem Minnesota integration were passed unanimously by the Park Nicollet Board on October 25, 1994. At the suggestion of rheumatologist Eric Schned, the Park Nicollet Management Committee recognized this integration by adopting a new name, Park Nicollet Clinic HealthSystem Minnesota.

Dr. Anthony Spagnolo, who came to Park Nicollet in 1985 as a member of the Shakopee Medical Center and who served on the HealthSystem Minnesota Bylaws Committee, said of the agreement, "We are doing this to put together a better, stronger, and more viable organization. I am impressed with how committed people are to make it work well." While acknowledging the sense of loss that would surely accompany the move, Reinertsen said after the vote, "We have gained something extraordinary."[98]

16

INTEGRATION AND COOPERATION

A WORKING SYSTEM

As Park Nicollet and Methodist Hospital were moving carefully toward the creation of "something extraordinary," the Twin Cities health care market continued its consolidation. In response to GroupCare/HealthPartners' successful bid for the BHCAG contract, the 500 independent physicians of Fairview Physicians Associates reorganized as a non-profit partner of Fairview Hospital and HealthCare Services in 1993.[99] That same year HealthPartners found the St. Paul Ramsey Medical Center ready and willing to be the first Minnesota hospital to be purchased by a health plan. The merger included the 200-physician Ramsey Clinic, the major providers of primary and specialty care at the University of Minnesota affiliated teaching hospital.[100] The two largest hospital groups, Health One and LifeSpan, merged in 1993 to form HealthSpan Health Systems with control of the Select Care PPO and 17 hospitals, including Abbott Northwestern in Minneapolis. In 1994 HealthSpan joined forces with the 550,000-member Medica HMO and formed Allina Health System.

The reorganization in Minnesota was going forward "at lightning speed," as James Reinertsen told the Physician Payment Review Commission in late 1993. Medical staffs were being restructured to meet the new market conditions "at the lowest specialty to primary care ratios practicable.

"The one asset that we have as an organization is our reputation. Once the patients have a perception that the care that they would receive here is questionable, we are out of the market. We're completely out of the market. The other thing is, they don't want to pay exorbitant costs for that care. For us to be competitive, we have to not only improve the quality of care we deliver and the service by which we deliver it, but we have to reduce the cost at the same time. Patients are turned away if you're too expensive, if you're rude, or if you're incompetent, so you can't do any one of those three things."

Richard Migliori, M.D.

HealthSystem Minnesota is currently at 50/50 and we are not recruiting specialists," Reinertsen told the commission. "At the same time, the existing primary care physicians have become precious and everyone is bidding for their loyalties."[101] This was raising the cost of primary care and accelerating a trend toward productivity-enhancing technologies which might allow the same number of physicians to serve more patients at a lower cost but with better outcomes. Park Nicollet, with more than seventy years of successfully managing change as a multispecialty group and now sharing an administrative structure with its primary hospital, was helping to push the market in this direction.

SERVICE, ACCESS, EFFICIENCY

Making the most of the new collaborative relationship with Methodist Hospital to meet the needs of cost and service, the internal medicine and family practice departments at Park Nicollet initiated a 24-hour in-hospital primary care service in January 1994. Four physicians during the day and one during evening and nighttime hours took care of all Park Nicollet patients and handled emergency care as needed. This system freed the majority of clinic physicians from daily hospital rounds. "The 24-Hour Service is more predictable for physicians, causing them to make fewer cancellations and have fewer behind-schedule days which makes for happier clinic patients," said Richard Freese, the internist who led the project.[102] A year later, a study by the Health Research Center, Park Nicollet Medical Foundation, confirmed that the in-hospital service was improving care and reducing costs. Patients noticed improvements as well, including less time waiting for appointments and easier phone scheduling.

Despite many clinical quality improvement successes, access continued to be a problem. The phone system was overwhelmed by the volume of calls that daily tied up all available circuits, and a new phone system installed in early 1995 only succeeded in compounding the problem. When patient surveys found 30 percent of patients ready to leave Park Nicollet if the phone problems weren't fixed, a cross-functional team of medical receptionists, computer specialists, nurses, and physicians was sent into action with a simple charge: fix the phones.

The solution that emerged used a combination of new computer technology and scheduling procedure changes to quickly route calls to the appropriate department or scheduler from a central number. Only after a telephone laboratory was installed in the internal medicine department to test the new system did the extent of the problem become clear. Patients had been waiting 354 seconds before a human voice answered, and 38 percent hung up in frustration before a human connection was made. By December 1995, with the new procedures implemented on a test basis, the waiting times were reduced to 60 seconds with only 9 percent hanging up before the call was completed. Service continues to improve toward the goal of 90 percent of calls answered within 30 seconds.

A key component of the new system is Phone Care, a nurse-staffed phone system that fields callers with acute symptoms. Phone Care was developed in cooperation with Blue Cross Blue Shield and fully implemented in January 1995. Operating 24 hours a day, 7 days a week, Phone Care staff uses a set of more than 120 computer-based guidelines to answer call-in questions from patients, offer home care options, and schedule appointments if needed. The guidelines are linked to the patient's medical record, and a chart note recording the transaction is automatically generated. The service succeeded in reducing the cost of service to the patient (fewer co-payments and fewer trips to the emergency room) and to the clinic (lower utilization, earlier diagnosis). The system has served "to help patients make decisions and provide care," said Sharon Reiter, R.N., manager of Phone Care.

BETTER OUTCOMES

The cancer centers at Methodist and Park Nicollet had attracted national recognition as statistical data on key quality indicators became more widely available. Methodist Hospital, for instance, had recorded 5-year survival rates for breast cancers that were 8 percent better than the national average, 4 percent better in lung cancers, 10 percent better in prostate cancers, and 9 percent better in colorectal cancer for the 1983 to 1990 reporting period.[103] In January 1995 oncologist Kathleen Ogle was selected to lead the new HealthSystem Minnesota Cancer Center. Patients continue to be seen at both locations, but administrative functions and technological resources are now combined to reduce duplication and to increase the quality and convenience of patient care.

The systems of care developed at Park Nicollet have produced equally impressive preventive care results. Screening and diagnostic programs at the new Jane Brattain Breast Diagnostic and Research Center had made it possible to find breast cancers in the two earliest stages 96 percent of the time, when it is most curable, compared to 75 percent nationally. Often cited as a quality indicator, regular screening for cervical cancer is exemplary at Park Nicollet. Records show that 91 percent of patients ages 18 to 75 had a current Pap smear on file—16 percent more than the state average among insured women.

The cardiac surgery program at Methodist, started in 1985 by Park Nicollet surgeons Hovald K. Helseth and Bjorn K. Monson, has an enviable record. Of 900 cardiac surgery programs surveyed in one study, Methodist Hospital ranked number one, showing a zero mortality rate for more than 100 Medicare patients in one year. No other cardiac surgery program in the Twin Cities was ranked in the top fifty programs nationwide.

Since 1989, when the Park Nicollet cardiothoracic surgery and cardiology departments were merged under the administrative leadership of Marjorie Canning, R.N., surgeons and internists have worked together to create a critical care team that is second to none. Using the continuous quality improvement process to develop a new protocol for thrombolytic therapy of acute myocardial infarction (heart attack) in 1995, HealthSystem Minnesota was able to increase the 30-day survival rate of heart attack patients from 91 to 97.5 percent, substantially above the national average. The excellent results didn't translate into higher costs. Methodist's coronary bypass surgery costs were shown to be about 5 percent below the state average, according to statistics compiled by the Minnesota Hospital Association.

BUILDING FOR THE FUTURE

While addressing questions of service and access, space needs continued to be a problem at Park Nicollet. It fell to John DeCoster, then director of real estate services, and his staff to find creative ways to accommodate the growing organization. The new Bloomington Clinic, designed to house the combined staffs of the two pre-merger Bloomington clinics in a new 40,000-square-foot colonial-style building at 98th and Normandale, was completed in April 1990. To finance further satellite construction, Park Nicollet, in cooperation with the City of St. Louis Park, successfully issued a $19.4 million Health Care Facilities Revenue Bond in October 1990. This financing led to the construction of the Imaging Center, which was installed in the Arneson Building on Excelsior (the original St. Louis Park Medical Center building), and new clinics on Cliff Road in Eagan (1991) and on the Carlson property at the intersection of I-394 and I-494 in Minnetonka (1992). The Ridgedale Clinic moved into the new Minnetonka building to serve the western suburbs.

In 1993 a two-story addition to the Burnsville Clinic, originally built by the Nicollet Clinic, more than doubled its size. At 93,500 square feet, the site was now twice the size of any of the other satellite offices, including the Blaisdell Avenue office which housed the Nicollet Clinic from 1960 until the merger in 1983. After a short pause in expansion efforts, the Shakopee Clinic began planning for a move to new, larger space adjacent to the new St. Francis Regional Medical Center. Opened in 1996, the new building includes a 20,000-square-foot Park Nicollet Clinic and an independent medical building, all directly connected to St. Francis Hospital.

TOWER PLACE

Perhaps the most significant building project undertaken by the organization in the 1990s was a major expansion of the old Northland building and site into a medical campus to be called Park Center. Environmental liability problems linked with the Beltline Pay Dump that underlay the site had been discovered in 1989. These problems, along with financial hurdles, had stalled negotiations for sale of the land and building by the Park Nicollet Medical Foundation back to Park Nicollet, which needed to hold title in order to issue the tax-free revenue bonds that would finance construction. This had caused Park Nicollet to postpone expansion of its central campus. Nevertheless, Park Nicollet and the foundation joined together in a voluntary remedial action plan (VRAP) to reclaim the site. This plan required long-term pumping of ground water from the dumpsite into the city sewers for treatment, special techniques and footings in any future construction to avoid disturbing the site, special methane venting, and regular monitoring of test wells for ground water contamination. This was the first plan of its kind in Minnesota, and the Minnesota Pollution Control Agency, which approved the plan in early 1993, won national recognition for its innovative reclamation efforts.[104]

With the VRAP in place, Park Nicollet and the foundation were able to come to a purchase agreement. In exchange for $1, the assumption of all related debt, all environmental liability above the $1 million dollars already allocated by the foundation to the VRAP, and a pledge by Park Nicollet to grant at least $1.883 million annually to the foundation, Park Nicollet would reassume ownership of its central clinical facilities. The transfer was initialed in June 1993 by Charles Jacobson, President and CEO of Park Nicollet, and Stuart Hanson, President of Park Nicollet Medical Foundation.

At the same time, a joint re-development project was outlined through a series of complex negotiations involving the St. Louis Park Economic Development Agency (EDA), Park Nicollet, the foundation, HealthSystem Minnesota, and Frauenshuh Companies (a private development company). Tower Place Project, so named for the water tower that had long stood at the corner of Highway 100 and Excelsior Boulevard, put forth a design that would dramatically reshape access to Park Nicollet by linking it directly to Excelsior Boulevard. The EDA agreed to contribute up to $6 million towards the VRAP, the Tower Place property development, and the construction of a 675-car city parking ramp on the site. Park Nicollet would take possession of the property, assume all future environmental liability and begin construction on two new clinical buildings.

Park Nicollet's building plans featured a two-story 55,000-square foot primary care clinic just to the west of the existing building. A new main entrance would welcome visitors through a sunny foyer protected by a translucent canopy. Family practice, internal medicine, and urgent care were slated to be located front row center in the new building, a visible reminder of the growing importance of primary care to managed care. The second planned building was a five-story surgery and ophthalmology center located along the west side of the entry drive south of the city parking ramp which would be connected to both buildings through heated walkways.

A separate agreement between Park Nicollet and the Frauenshuh Company allowed the development company to build and manage a retail, restaurant, and movie center on the southwest corner of the property. A long-term option on this commercial land was included to reserve space for future expansion of the Park Nicollet campus.

In April 1993 the Tower Place Redevelopment Agreement was signed by all parties. HealthSystem Minnesota, as the parent organization, approved the formation of an obligated group, including HSM, Methodist Hospital, and Park Nicollet, to issue the bonds needed to finance construction. A total of $225 million in Health Care Facilities Revenue Bonds were sold on September 1, 1993.[105]

Ground-breaking took place on September 22, 1993, and construction continued through the winter and spring. Announcing the start of construction, Charles Jacobson said "the expansion of our campus is a symbol of Park Nicollet's commitment to the highest quality health care and service. We are building a new model for health care—one that is primary care based and community oriented."[106] The project was completed, and 1,300 community members and 200 volunteers celebrated the grand opening on April 25, 1995.

INSTITUTE FOR RESEARCH AND EDUCATION

As affiliation talks that led to the formation of HealthSystem Minnesota progressed, Park Nicollet Medical Foundation chose to remain apart from the discussions. As an integral but very independent part of Park Nicollet, the foundation was committed to preserving its independent status. Once the HSM structure was in place, Jim Reinertsen met with Stuart Hanson, president of the foundation, and James Toscano, executive vice president. The interchange was "upbeat, enthusiastic and optimistic," according to Toscano.[107] "I asked for the hardest thing I could think of—that HSM change its mission to include a commitment to additional core values in research and education, and Reinertsen said 'yes, I've been thinking we need to do that,'" Toscano recalled.

HSM needed the foundation's expertise and reputation for independent, high-quality science-based research and education programming to add value to its health care services. The foundation needed close ties to its primary medical staff and clinical laboratory. "Interested, engaged, motivated physicians are critical to the work of [the foundation], which itself seeks to foster ideas, curiosity and enthusiasms and transform these into research and education programs," the foundation's proposal to HSM stated.[108] After a year of detailed preparations, the Park Nicollet Medical Foundation board was ready to join HealthSystem Minnesota as a self-governing subsidiary operating as the Institute for Research and Education. Responsible for research, education, and research and development programs for all of HSM, the institute officially began operations on January 1, 1996.

STATEMENT OF STRATEGIC INTENT

The Institute for Research and Education will create, evaluate and disseminate knowledge for transforming, organizing and financing health care and other systems to improve patient health care, population health and public accountability.

Institute Divisions Prosper

The Health Research Center, under the leadership of Jinnet Fowles, Ph.D., Renner Anderson, M.D., and Margaret Healey, Ph.D., brings professionalism in scientific scrutiny to the institute's growing national reputation as a research organization. Research projects in ambulatory care, quality and consumer choice in managed care, outcomes, and risk management were all completed in the early 1990s, including work by Dave Knutson, Director of Health Systems Studies, which involved large surveys of BHCAG's pediatric and senior populations.

The International Diabetes Center (IDC) continues to flourish as an international source of information and expe-

"The role of the foundation I think is central to the success of this organization. We've got to continue to learn how to do things better, cheaper, and with better service in shorter cycle times. The foundation's key strength is its ability to help us do the research that's necessary to answer the question: Are we in fact doing it better, cheaper, and with better service."

Richard Migliori, M.D.

rience in diabetes research and education under the direction of endocrinologist Richard Bergenstal, who succeeded IDC founder Donnell Etzwiler just prior to Etzwiler's retirement in November 1996. Headed by Roger Mazze, Ph.D., the Staged Diabetes Management™ (SDM) program was developed and published by the IDC in 1995. The program offers a series of diagnostic and treatment decision paths that studies have shown improve outcomes, decrease practice variation, and lower costs. Backed by training and group strategies designed to support implementation, the program has been adopted by 27 sites in Minnesota through the financial support of the state Lions association. More than 100 SDM sites have been established in the United States, and through the IDC's work as a World Health Organization Collaborating Center in diabetes, the program has been adapted for use in seven foreign countries, including Japan, Brazil, Russia, and Poland. Besides SDM, the IDC publishes and distributes consumer books such as *Fast Food Facts*, *Exchanges for All Occasions*, and *Managing Type II Diabetes*, along with patient education materials such as *My Food Plan* and the *Type II Diabetes Prevention Pyramids*.

The Health Education Center, headed by Paul Terry, Ph.D., continues to develop health education programs and to add successful titles to its publications catalog. *A Primer for Prevention*, *Living with Asthma: A Practical Guide to Understanding and Managing Asthma*, and *Living with ADHD: A Practical Guide to Coping with Attention Deficit Hyperactivity Disorder* are just a few of the titles that have achieved wide distribution. *Well Advised: A Practical Guide to Everyday Health Decisions*, edited by Paul Terry with Park Nicollet physicians David Abelson and Allan Kind, was published by Mosby-Great Productions and is available at bookstores around the country. The *Activity Pyramid*, a learning tool created by Jane Nordstrom, M.A., has sold hundreds of thousands of copies to businesses nationwide. The Health Education Center received the C. Everett

Koop National Health Award in 1994 for its continuing success in demonstrating cost savings through health education.[109]

THE NEXT 75 YEARS

Seventy-five years after its establishment as a private practice, multispecialty group, Park Nicollet has grown to include nearly 400 physicians, 170 clinical professionals, and a total staff of more than 1800 who provide care to more than 15 percent of the Twin Cities metropolitan population. The vertical integration of the physician group and the hospital has created opportunities to reorganize the combined management team according to the patients' experience of care without competition for resources within the system, and to develop new technologies and services to complement the mission of the combined organization.

The vision of integrating primary, secondary, and tertiary care into a system that can be managed for the benefit of the patient has been nurtured within the collective organizational culture since the Nicollet Clinic founders first contemplated the purchase of a hospital in the 1920s. It was evident when a new generation of physicians created a new model that incorporated prepaid care into private group practice in 1972. It then became a reality when Park Nicollet and Methodist Hospital formed a new alliance that became HealthSystem Minnesota in 1993. It is a living vision, one which changes and is changed by society and by economic realities. But most importantly the vision is changed by the people who get up each day thinking of new ways to improve the processes of care.

The challenge for the future, Reinertsen says, is to succeed in making HealthSystem Minnesota an indispensable care system. "We want our patients, our community, our business purchasers and our health plan partners to regard

James Reinertsen and Rodney Dueck introduced the Quality Diamond in 1995 to graphically reinforce the core values of the organization and to help keep these values uppermost in the minds of the entire staff. The four points of the diamond represent Care, Joy, Service, and Stewardship. Rooted in the Park Nicollet continuous quality improvement program, the Quality Diamond provides focus for an ongoing dialogue throughout the organization. It urges each member of HealthSystem Minnesota to continually ask the question: Is this the best process, policy, work style, or habit to support excellence in care, superb customer service, real stewardship, and lasting joy in work? Reinertsen's challenge is: If the answer is no, then we have work to do.

HealthSystem Minnesota as essential," Reinertsen said. "To become truly indispensable, we must improve our patients' perception of our service, improve our efficiency and productivity as a system, consolidate our market position, and tell the story of our exceptional quality at every opportunity."[110]

Chapter 12

1 Blue Cross and Blue Shield of Minnesota, *The Blue Cross and Blue Shield of Minnesota Story: A Sixty-Year History* (St. Paul: BCBS, 1993), 78.
2 Glen D. Nelson, "The Minneapolis-St. Paul Experience," in James R. Gay and Barbara J. Sax Jacobs, eds., *Competition in the Marketplace: Health Care in the 1980s* (New York: SP Medical and Scientific Books, 1982), 57.
3 Roger Asplin, Administrator's Annual Report, St. Louis Park Medical Center, 1975.
4 Tom Hobban, interview with Emily Freidman and Jim Hare, April 5, 1994.
5 "Citizens League Urges Twin Cities Cut 4,000 Beds," *Minneapolis Tribune*, September 20, 1977, A1.
6 Minutes of Shakopee Medical Center, June 11, 1984.
7 Glen Nelson, written responses to interview with author, January 1, 1995.
8 Minutes of the St. Louis Park Medical Center Board, April 7, 1981.
9 The SHARE Clinic and Health Plan, despite its weak showing in 1980, continued its rapid growth, enrolling 100,000 members by 1984. In 1991 it merged with Physicians Health Plan to create Medica.
10 James Stolhanske, Minutes of the St. Louis Park Medical Center Board, December 7, 1982.
11 David Jensen, Minutes of the Medcenter Health Plan Board, January 13, 1983.
12 Glen Nelson, Annual Report of St. Louis Park Medical Center, 1982.
13 Letter from Earl Young to Glen Nelson, February 24, 1983.
14 Eitel Hospital, Abbott Northwestern Hospital, and the Sister Kenny Institute became the founding members of Lifespan in 1982.
15 Theresa Baker (Ryan), Annual Report of St. Louis Park Medical Center, 1983.
16 Arthur Ide, Loren Vorlicky, and many others have used this phrase.
17 Glen Nelson, Annual Report of Park Nicollet Medical Center, 1983.
18 Thomas Recht, Annual Report of the Nicollet Clinic, 1983.
19 Glen Nelson, Annual Report of Park Nicollet Medical Center, 1983.
20 Ibid.

Chapter 13

21 John K. Iglehart, "Health Policy Report: The Twin Cities Medical Marketplace," *New England Journal of Medicine* 311(August 2, 1984): 343, 346.
22 Robert Wood Johnson Foundation, *The Transformation of the U.S. Health Care Market*, December 1995, 4.
23 Paul Starr, *The Social Transformation of American Medicine* (New York: Basic Books, 1982), 428.
24 Richard Reeves, "The Corporate Transformation of Medicine in Minnesota: The First of a Series: The Accelerating Industrialization of Health Care in the Twin Cities," *Minnesota Medicine* 67(May 1984): 251.
25 "Technology Provides New Avenues for Exports, *Star Tribune*, January 5, 1986, 1D.
26 Glen Nelson, written communication with author, August 17, 1994.
27 Loren Vorlicky, interview with author, October 5, 1994.
28 Glen Nelson, written communication with author, August 17, 1994.
29 Reeves, "The Corporate Transformation of Medicine in Minnesota," 309.
30 David Jensen, interview with author, April 24, 1995, and Minutes of MedCenters Health Plan, March 16, 1984.
31 Glen Nelson, Minutes of the Park Nicollet Medical Center Board, April 24, 1984.
32 Glen Nelson, Minutes of the Park Nicollet Medical Center Board, July 11, 1984.
33 Minutes of the MedCenters Health Plan Board, July 23, 1984.
34 Annual Report of American MedCenters, 1984.
35 David Lilly, memorandum to Park Nicollet Medical Center staff, July 20, 1984.
36 Ibid.
37 Glen Nelson, Minutes of the Park Nicollet Medical Center Board, August 28, 1984.
38 "AMED Announces Earnings," *What's News?* May 10, 1985, 1.
39 Glen Nelson, written comments to author, January 18, 1995.
40 Final Report of the Park Nicollet Medical Center Task Force on Access to Care, June 1983.
41 William Telleen, Minutes of the Park Nicollet Medical Center Board, July 25, 1989.
42 Annual Report of the Home Health Care Department, 1984.
43 Paul Batalden, Annual Report of Park Nicollet Medical Center, 1984.
44 Ibid.

45 Minutes of the Park Nicollet Medical Center Board, April 22, 1986.
46 Minutes of the Park Nicollet Medical Center Board, January 10, 1984; Roger Upson, Minutes of Executive Committee, Park Nicollet Medical Center Board, April 11, 1984; Roger Upson, Minutes of the Park Nicollet Medical Center Board, June 25, 1985.
47 Max Boller, Minutes of Executive Committee, Park Nicollet Medical Center Board, February 14, 1984.
48 Glen Nelson, President's Annual Report, Park Nicollet Medical Center, 1985.
49 McKinsey & Company, "Organizing for Success in a Changing Industry Environment: PNMC/AMED/Methodist Hospital," December 17, 1985, 7.
50 Glen Nelson, President's Annual Report, Park Nicollet Medical Center, 1985.

Chapter 14
51 James Reinertsen, President's Annual Report, Park Nicollet Medical Center, 1986.
52 James Reinertsen, "'Patients First' Begins in January," *MedNews*, January 16, 1987, 1.
53 Carol Hersman, "'Patients First' Begins in January," *MedNews*, January 16, 1987, 1.
54 Gamble Task Force on Physician Management Structure, McKinsey: Final Summary Report of Actions, February 1988, 11.
55 Joseph Mitlyng, personal communication with author, February 16, 1995.
56 MedCenters acceptance of this argument was due in part to the fact that at the time Blue Cross Blue Shield's AWARE Gold program was actively recruiting Park Nicollet Medical Center, threatening the long-standing, exclusive relationship the medical center maintained with MedCenters. On August 22, 1986, medical center board minutes record an offer to MedCenters to forego participation in AWARE Gold in return for a shift in capitation payments from the end of the month to the beginning of the month.
57 Loren Vorlicky, personal communication with author, September 1, 1995.
58 President's Annual Report, Park Nicollet Medical Center, 1986.
59 Judith Yates Borger, "Tube Test, PN Tries TV," *Corporate Report* (April 1987): 39.
60 James Reinertsen, Minutes of the Park Nicollet Medical Center Board, April 22, 1986.
61 James Reinertsen, Minutes of the Park Nicollet Medical Center Board, February 16, 1987.

62 Richard Reeves, "Corporate Transformation of Medicine in Minnesota: The View From Eagan," *Minnesota Medicine* 69(March 1986): 115.
63 The decision was not unanimous. Max Boller and Robert Olson voted against joining AWARE Gold and William Schoenwetter voted for arbitration.
64 Joseph Mitlyng, Minutes of the Park Nicollet Medical Center Board, August 25, 1987.
65 Arbitration Order, Edward J. Petras et al., January 21, 1988, also the Majority Memorandum attachment.
66 Cease and Desist Order, Minnesota Commissioner of Health, January 29, 1988.
67 Joseph Mitlyng, Minutes of the Park Nicollet Medical Center Board, May 16, 1989.
68 Joseph Mitlyng, Monthly Operations Report, Minutes of the Park Nicollet Medical Center Board, April 11, 1989.
69 W. Edwards Deming, *Out of the Crisis* (Cambridge, Mass.: Massachusetts Institute of Technology, Center for Advanced Engineering Study, 1982), 199. (An abbreviated list.)
70 Donald Berwick, "Improving Quality in Medical Care," *Park Nicollet Medical Foundation Bulletin* 34(1990, no.1): 16.
71 Rodney Dueck, "The Power and Principles of CQI," *Park Nicollet Medical Center Bulletin* 36(1992, no. 2): 87.
72 James Reinertsen, Annual President's Report, Park Nicollet Medical Center, 1990.
73 Dueck, "The Power and Principles of CQI," 91.
74 "Our Mission Statement," Park Nicollet Medical Center, June 1990, as it appeared in "Park Nicollet Medical Center's Continuous Quality Improvement Process," revised, March 1991.
75 Minutes of a meeting on November 6, 1984, report that Glen Nelson and Paul Batalden urged "all deliberate speed in creating a 501(c)(3) holding company to coordinate operation of the related organizations; until then the organizations need to be functionally interlocked, with Nelson as the integrating link." There were, however, no more references in the minutes to further progress along this line.
76 *MedNews*, June 30, 1989.
77 William Telleen, Minutes of the Park Nicollet Medical Center Board Minutes, August 22, 1989.
78 Minutes, Special Meeting of the Park Nicollet Medical Center Board, January 25, 1985.
79 Minutes of the Park Nicollet Medical Center Board, May 14, 1985.
80 Douglas W. Fenstermaker et al., "Provider Downsizing and Restructuring: 'How to Make Less More,'" Conference Proceedings, Minneapolis, November 16, 1993.

81 "Park Nicollet Medical Center: Year in Review, 1991"; Park Nicollet Medical Center Board approved agreement on November 21, 1991, according to audit report for 1990-91.

82 Douglas A. Shaw and Thomas W. Hobban, "Twin Cities Health Care Mergers, Acquisitions, and Affiliations: Implications for Independent Physician Practices," *Minnesota Medicine* 75(September 1991): 24-31.

Chapter 15

83 *Methodist and Park Nicollet News*, no. 3, March 28, 1992.

84 *Methodist and Park Nicollet News*, no. 1, January 3 1992.

85 Methodist Associates was the employed physicians' group within Methodist Hospital.

86 "Minnesota: A Great State of Health" was coined in the early 1980s by James Toscano and Patty Newman and promoted by the Minnesota Department of Economic Development.

87 Shaw and Hobban, "Twin Cities Health Care Mergers," 24.

88 Ron Winslow, "Strong Medicine, Employers' Attack on Health Costs Spurs Change in Minnesota," *Wall Street Journal*, February 26, 1993, A1.

89 Shaw and Hobban, "Twin Cities Health Care Mergers," 292.

90 "MedCenters, Group Health Partnership Announced," *Star Tribune*, April 25, 1992, A1.

91 Shaw and Hobban, "Twin Cities Health Care Mergers," 27.

92 Gordon Slovut, "Big Firms Join in Health Plan," *Star Tribune*, July 1, 1992, 1B.

93 Ibid.

94 James Reinertsen, "What Does System Thinking Have to Do with HealthSystem Minnesota?" (Annual Report to Board of Directors, HealthSystem Minnesota, May 3, 1994).

95 Ibid.

96 Ibid.

97 Charles Jacobson, Administrative Update, Park Nicollet Board meeting, February 3, 1994.

98 Anthony Spagnolo and James Reinertsen, Administrative Update, Park Nicollet Board meeting, October 25, 1994.

Chapter 16

99 Anita J. Slomski, "Business to doctors: Show us you're doing it right," *Medical Economics*, August 9, 1993, 70.

100 Tom Majeski, "Strong Rx for Change: Competition," *St. Paul Pioneer Press*, November 13, 1994, 1.

101 James L. Reinertsen, MD, "Health System Reform, Marketplaces, and Physician Manpower: Public Statement to Physician Payment Review Commission," February 7, 1996.

102 "New 24-Hour Hospital Service improves care and increases efficiency," *Insights*, September 1995, 1.

103 HSM Annual report, citing SEER Cancer Statistics Review, 1973 - 1991, National Cancer Institute, NIH Pub No. 94-2789, 1994.

104 *MedNews*, October 1994, 4.

105 *Finance Highlights,* December 1993, Administrative Update.

106 Charles, Jacobson, M.D., Quote from "For Your Health," internal publication, 1993.

107 James Toscano (Internal memo, Park Nicollet Medical Foundation, September 8, 1994).

108 "Exploring a New Relationship Between Park Nicollet Medical Foundation and HealthSystem Minnesota," (Internal document, September 8, 1996).

109 Park Nicollet Medical Foundation 1994 Annual Report, 8.

110 James Reinertsen, "Becoming an Indispensable Care System: A conversation with James L. Reinertsen, M.D., *Insights*, January 1996, 4.

Colophon

This book was set in Caslon and Copperplate types with Caslon ornaments and printed on Sterling Web gloss and Sterling Web matte papers.